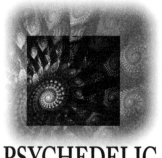

PSYCHEDELIC
HEALING

"*Psychedelic Healing* is full of knowledge and wisdom, psychologically sophisticated, and up-to-date. It contains important lessons for those wishing to work with psychedelic plants and substances, which are powerful and tricky tools for accessing the psyche. Neal Goldsmith makes a well-reasoned plea for society to use them once again because they are important tools for healing inside, healing relationships, and healing society. I enjoyed his speculation about the post-postmodern synthesis of tribal and modern. Written bravely and with open eyes, this is an important, mature book"

JEREMY NARBY, PH.D., AUTHOR OF *THE COSMIC SERPENT* AND
CO-EDITOR OF *SHAMANS THROUGH TIME*

"*Psychedelic Healing* offers the reader a wondrous journey, capturing within one volume a guide for the use of psychedelics by therapists and patients as well as a contemporary summation of relevant research and points of history. Goldsmith bravely goes where few dare to tread, especially in his autobiographical vignettes that make clear how what is learned through psychedelic-assisted therapy can usefully be applied and integrated into everyday life. This book is highly recommended to anyone interested in learning how psychedelics may contribute to a healthier, richer, and more rewarding life rather than just assuming that these substances must be categorized as drugs of abuse. There is more to these substances than their pejorative categorizations within a Drug War: *Psychedelic Healing* offers an easy-to-read path to these deeper waters."

JOHN H. HALPERN, M.D., ASSISTANT PROFESSOR OF
PSYCHIATRY, HARVARD MEDICAL SCHOOL

"Neal Goldsmith is one of the leading architects of the emerging paradigm of psychedelic therapy. In this book he shares the personal story of his own process of growth and transformation as both a drug policy analyst and a psychotherapist and boldly calls for the acceptance and integration of psychedelics into psychiatry and society as the powerful catalysts for self-exploration and healing that they are."

DENNIS MCKENNA, PH.D., ASSISTANT PROFESSOR,
CENTER FOR SPIRITUALITY AND HEALING,
UNIVERSITY OF MINNESOTA

"Neal Goldsmith's comprehensive, wise, and timely guide explores the impact of psychedelics throughout history and today at the level of the individual, the society, and the collective consciousness. *Psychedelic Healing* addresses salient theoretical questions pertinent to policy, therapy, spirituality, and philosophy and offers a bountiful harvest of hard-earned insights to every reader interested in the transformative power of psychedelics. Neal has made a major contribution to ensuring the continued expansion of the psychedelic research renaissance. *Psychedelic Healing* will enable motivated readers to work more effectively to create a world where the mature use of psychedelics for spiritual, psychological, and medical purposes is both accepted and appreciated."

RICK DOBLIN, PH.D, EXECUTIVE DIRECTOR,
MULTIDISCIPLINARY ASSOCIATION FOR PSYCHEDELIC STUDIES

"In this lively and provocative book, Neal M. Goldsmith, Ph.D., makes the case for a 'Psychedelic Renaissance,' one in which LSD-type substances would be rescheduled in the United States, permitting their applications in psychotherapy and medicine. *Psychedelic Healing* presents considerable evidence from the research and clinical literature, as well as from Goldsmith's own experiences, that psychedelics can relieve pain, change personality, foster spiritual growth, and promote community harmony. After reading this book, many of his readers will be persuaded that this renaissance cannot come a day too soon!"

STANLEY KRIPPNER, PH.D., ALAN WATTS PROFESSOR
OF PSYCHOLOGY, SAYBROOK UNIVERSITY,
AND COAUTHOR OF *PERSONAL MYTHOLOGY*

"Written with personal warmth and passionate engagement, *Psychedelic Healing* makes a compelling case for the medical and social benefits of a therapy practice that encompasses substance-induced experiences of transcendence. With scrupulous care, Neal Goldsmith explores the great promise of this reemerging field, while proposing a path forward that avoids the mistakes made a generation ago. This book is valuable reading for those who would like to see a crucial new chapter open in consciousness studies and the mental health field."

DANIEL PINCHBECK, AUTHOR OF *BREAKING OPEN THE HEAD*

"What a brave and wonderful book! Neal Goldsmith beautifully integrates personal experience and reflections with thoughtful analysis of psychedelics: their history, prohibition and regulation, and potential for transforming our psyches, spirits, and lives."

ETHAN A. NADELMANN, J.D., PH.D, EXECUTIVE DIRECTOR
OF THE DRUG POLICY ALLIANCE

"A wonderful blend of psychedelic history. Goldsmith has written a radical, wise, and compassionate rethinking of the nature and purpose of psychotherapy. This is the direction psychology needs to go in order to stay relevant and valuable."

JAMES FADIMAN PH.D., AUTHOR OF *THE PSYCHEDELIC EXPLORERS GUIDE* AND *PERSONALITY AND PERSONAL GROWTH*

"A thoroughly researched and engaging discussion of psychedelic-assisted psychotherapy, profiling not just the drugs, but many luminaries in the psychedelic research field. Goldsmith emphasizes the importance of set, setting, and ritual on outcome. By chronicling his own growth and transformation he answers the question, 'Is fundamental personality change possible?' with an emphatic 'Yes!'"

JULIE HOLLAND, M.D., EDITOR OF *ECSTASY: THE COMPLETE GUIDE* AND *THE POT BOOK: A COMPLETE GUIDE TO CANNABIS*

"When we look back at the extraordinary cultural transformations of the past forty years, there is one ingredient in the recipe of social change that is consistently and inexplicably expunged from the record. And that is the fact that countless thousands, indeed millions, of young at some point in their lives lay prostrate before the gates of awe having taken a psychedelic. Neal Goldsmith's insightful book suggests that perhaps we might do well by doing the same."

WADE DAVIS, AWARD-WINNING ANTHROPOLOGIST, ETHNOBOTANIST, FILMMAKER, AUTHOR, AND PHOTOGRAPHER

"Neal Goldsmith's comprehensive analysis of the healing power of psychedelics puts the medical, spiritual, and legal status of these soul medicines in a passionate, well-informed voice."

ALEX GREY, AUTHOR OF *SACRED MIRRORS* AND *TRANSFIGURATIONS*

"*Psychedelic Healing* is a comprehensive contextualized guide for harnessing psychedelics to assist in personal evolution. Neal Goldsmith introduces you to all the key players at this exciting moment in the long history of human interaction with psychedelic plants. Goldsmith's clinical yet revealing and accessible narrative is as reassuring as it is instructional. Not since *The Tibetan Book of the Dead* has there been such a useful companion to the amazing array of spiritual medicines that are nature's gift to humanity."

ALLAN BADINER, ADJUNCT PROFESSOR AT THE CALIFORNIA INSTITUTE OF INTEGRAL STUDIES, CONTRIBUTING EDITOR AT *TRICYCLE*, AND EDITOR OF *ZIG ZAG ZEN: BUDDHISM AND PSYCHEDELICS*

This book is dedicated to three groups of courageous individuals.

First, the shamans, sadhus, curendaros, and ayahuasceros who over millennia developed and kept alive the spiritual use of visionary plants and who—once Western civilization came to power—were often demonized and persecuted for their dedication to this window to our perfection.

Second, the researchers and therapists who came next and over the past century have worked to understand, translate, and reintegrate psychedelics into Western civilization. These dedicated, tenacious professionals were often marginalized in their chosen fields, sometimes treated as outcasts or even criminals, all because they saw and hoped to share the profound importance of these incomparable psychospiritual tools.

Third, the research subjects, clinical patients, and ordinary citizens who strove to benefit from these deeply grounding, healing, and transformative medicine-sacraments, often suffering great pain, as society struggled to intelligently access, maturely use, and effectively incorporate the power and the beauty of the psychedelic experience.

I am grateful to these brave pioneers for enabling this book to be written.

A Note on the Use of Psychedelics

Psychedelics are the most powerful psychiatric medicine (and spiritual sacrament) known to humanity. They offer great promise to Western psychiatry as clinical tools for treating medical disorders. Of even greater significance is their contribution to normal human development throughout the life cycle. In fact, the very power of this most powerful class of substances has also brought about a grave lessening of the quality of life for many. Especially for the unprepared, psychedelics can engender unexpected, intense, and unpleasant experiences such as temporary psychotic breaks, and they can trigger permanent mental illness in the predisposed. Currently, there are no formally trained psychedelic therapists legally permitted to practice, and the available underground (illegal) psychedelic therapists are of uncertain and variable quality. To make matters worse, due to their prohibition, the doses and purity of psychedelic substances bought illegally are generally unknown to the consumer. Consequently, until a time when the quality of the therapy and the dose and purity of these substances can be known, I recommend that those interested in the effects of psychedelics do their homework, take these intriguing substances ONLY in certified research projects (see www.maps.org/research for a list), and actively work to change the drug laws and to encourage government funding for psychedelic research.

CONTENTS

WHY THIS BOOK MATTERS

John H. Halpern, M.D., Harvard Medical School

In ancient times, psychedelic plants were venerated as sacred sacraments and tools of divination and healing. Even to the present day, we find them employed as *entheogens:* "manifesting God within." Traditional and religious use of entheogens thrive in many cultures, for example: iboga in western Africa, ayahuasca in the Amazon basin, psilocybin-containing mushrooms and *Salvia divinorum* in southern Mexico, and mescaline-containing cacti in Peru and North America. Reviled in the "modern" Western world, these substances were (and are) revered in the shamanic world, and their spiritual "goodness" is inexorably reaching out to the rest of us. Although the Ghost Dance was successfully stamped out in the nineteenth century, the syncretic peyote religion took root pan-tribally across the United States and Canada.

Today, the Native American Church is the largest faith among Native Americans. The syncretic ayahuasca faiths (primarily the Santo Daime and União do Vegetal, or UDV) have welcomed congregants beyond native peoples and are legally recognized within their Latin American countries of origin. Indeed, Santo Daime and UDV have membership around the globe and are now protected in the United States. Some members feel that these "medicines" are choosing today to reveal themselves to the greater world to raise the consciousness necessary for saving our souls and planet. The Christian missionaries put their best into bringing these peoples of faith to a Western vision; how interesting that, in return, now the primary experience of these psycho-active sacraments offers communion with the Creator for a Western world that is increasingly secularized and desacralized.

While Western nations cling to the assumption that these substances are primarily drugs of abuse that can promote mental illness and social upheaval, what does this say about the four hundred thousand members of the Native American Church who happily and healthfully venerate peyote as their holy sacrament? Long before there was a Canada or a United States, their ancestors knew these experiences were safe within their proper use and potentially harmful in their abuse. The Western skeptic's perspective may be locked into a doubt that originates in ethnocentrism, an over-reliance on a scientific model, or a simple fear of the unfamiliar and unknown. Yet the world is maturing in favor of a more accepting vision. The use of peyote in the United States and Canada is restricted to native peoples out of treaty obligations to protect and uphold their traditional cultural practices: for them, peyote is their Eucharist, their Holy Sacrament, the flesh of God given for their specific betterment. It is a vision that protects, loves, and heals. History is replete with examples of our taking native lands, their way of life; and there will long be fears that we will take their Holy Medicine from them, too. But, in fact, native peoples were the first "plugged in" to a World Consciousness. Those who assumed the "backward savage" will give up their ways for our presumed superior power, technologies, and education, instead will find that systems do get co-opted in both directions. Tobacco is an important tool for prayer throughout the Western Hemisphere among native peoples, but the Europeans stripped tobacco from its holy purpose. In its routine daily abuse, tobacco cigarettes kill. As Schedule I drugs of abuse, the "hallucinogens" can and do bring harm and are labeled dangerous and unpredictable. Is this so for Native American Church members? Is this what we assume for those who have a legal "exemption"? Or is their use a message—a teaching—about ourselves, about who we are and who are meant to be, about the transformation of ourselves that is a natural unfolding that we might otherwise ignore or only have a subtle awareness of, because it is so basic to what it means to be a human being?

If we move to the psychiatric model, we find these substances defined by single words such as *psychotogen, psychotomimetic,* and *mysticomimetic,* to *psychedelic, hallucinogen,* or *entheogen.* The revelation of the inner world is a risk—to see our inexperience at recognizing our primal self. It is far safer to shelve these substances as unpredictable and not pause to consider what it means if the unpredictability is predictable. If you dismiss and reject on faith that there can be something "real" or of value for you within what are supposed to be drugs only of abuse, without any benefits, then you will also walk away assured that there is no reason to think for yourself. Oppose this model and society is supposed to ignore you, because there just cannot be any consistent means for induction of sacred consciousness. If we understand these substances to be only "drugs of abuse" and harm, with rarely experienced but endlessly propagandized flashbacks and worse (such as psychosis in those who are predisposed), then where is the confidence to appreciate that these may also be special tools for introspection, healing, and religious/ spiritual expression? Where is the guidance that can open our eyes to what are also "humility agonists" that "narcissistilyse" through layers of defenses piled up as we age?

I encourage you to take in this book as one that is such a guide. The real guide for you is the one you write for yourself. Dr. Goldsmith offers you his, and, if you read it carefully, you will gain a method that you can modify as you see fit for your personal discovery, with or without ingesting any substance. Read this volume as a unified story: Dr. Goldsmith bravely offers himself as an illustration of what psychotherapy and insight is possible with psychedelics. Consider this book as a consultation from a specialist: you will be introduced to the history of psychedelics, key researchers and other figures, lessons on safety, change, and psychology, examples "in the field," and even a very special suggested reading list!

This book matters because it offers a systematic explanation of the power of these substances and how they may be harnessed for mental health, personal growth, and spiritual nourishment. In the wrong hands (Charlie Manson and the Aum Shirikio cult come to mind), these are aides of indoctrination and megalomaniacism. C. S. Jung found his archetypes of synchronicity through his exploration of his inner world, but hesitated to share his Red Book of personal insight for fear it might be misunderstood as a mescaline-like phantasmic allegorical. In synchronous timing with the publication of Jung's precious personal vision, Dr. Goldsmith presents his own Red Book of self discovery and organizes it into a useful roadmap to the mystery within each of us—of who we are and why. Each of us is different: this is the unpredictability so much harped on by detractors of entheogens without awareness of predictabilitity—the reliability by which we can grow and accept and even alter who we are and to come closer to the sacred goal of who we are meant to become. There are no shortcuts, but with the proper digesting of Dr. Goldsmith's efforts within these pages you may just recognize that you possess some blinking lights directing you to put your foot onto your path and to behold the wonders and simple pleasures of your life, as the journey of enlightenment that takes you toward your destiny.

JOHN H. HALPERN, M.D.

Dr. John Halpern is an assistant professor of psychiatry at Harvard Medical School and director of the Laboratory for Integrative Psychiatry at McLean Hospital in Belmont, Massachusetts. His research projects include evaluating cognitive performance of MDMA users and nonusers in the Southwest as well as researching the effects of MDMA-assisted psychotherapy as an experimental treatment for advanced-stage cancer patients. Dr. Halpern has authored or coauthored several primary reference medical textbook chapters on hallucinogen use and abuse and is a recipient of grant support from private foundations as well as from the National Institute on Drug Abuse, National Institutes of Health.

ACKNOWLEDGMENTS

I would like to gratefully acknowledge the many individuals who have contributed to producing this book.

Several individuals (listed here alphabetically) spent valuable time reading and commenting on earlier drafts of this book. I thank: my friend and a true hero, attorney Richard Glen Boire, founder of the Center for Cognitive Liberty and Ethics and role model for all those with a passion for rational drug policy; my dear friend Jessi Daichman, whose grounded spirituality and unwavering encouragement contributed fundamentally to my intention to create a book dedicated solely to the betterment of my readers; my dear friend and colleague Rick Doblin, founder and executive director of the Multidisciplinary Association for Psychedelic Studies (MAPS)—who one day will have a book written about him and the inexhaustible dedication and energy he has brought to the mission of reintroducing psychedelics into our culture; John Halpern, brilliant Harvard research psychiatrist and friend, who has shared his ideas and helped me immensely by writing a fact-filled foreword that has added substantively to this book; my gentle friend and brilliant intellectual sparring partner, Dan Merkur; Tom Roberts, who contributed to the very existence of this book by inviting me to write for his textbook *Psychedelic Medicine* the chapter upon which this book was based; Ed Rosenfeld, my dear friend of twenty-five years who first introduced me to the scholarly literature and cultural lore on psychedelics; my brother-in-law, dear friend, and extraordinary scholar and spiritual adept, Carleton Schade, who lovingly spurred me to create the very best book I had in me; and Richard Yensen, whose unbending ethics and continuing friendship have been a model to me and many others in this field. I thank each of you for contributing your time, intelligence, and love to my project.

I would also like to acknowledge the staff of my publisher, Inner Traditions, for their unwavering support—and patience—as my proposal became a manuscript and that manuscript became this book. In particular, I thank my acquisitions editor, Jon Graham, for bringing me into the Inner Traditions fold, managing editor Jeanie Levitan, for her gracious kindness as I began my relationship with Inner Traditions, and especially project editor Chanc VanWinkle Orzell and copy editor Lynne Ertle, whose combined insight, attention to detail, and breadth of experience literally transformed this book from a collection of heartfelt insights and ideas into a professional, readable, and publishable volume.

Finally, I would like to acknowledge the loving support of my family during the creation of this book. My parents, Shirley and Victor Goldsmith, whose dedication to education, scholarship, language, logic, honesty, and effort molded my mind and heart in ways that can be felt on every page. My wife, Debra, who has from the beginning supported my growth as I pursued my interest in psychedelic scholarship—an endeavor still not fully acceptable to many and so not without negative consequences, which she accepted with grace. Finally, my fine twelve-year-old son, Jared, who sacrificed in ways he is not even aware of as I spent time on this book that could have been spent with him. I hope he will read this book one day with a blossoming mind, an open heart, and pride in his father's intention.

PREFACE

Writing this book was a profound experience for me, and I hope that it will be a profound experience for you, the reader, as well. This book explores the biggest themes in society—spirituality, Cartesian duality, existential reality, psychological transformation, survival, and sustainability—yet it also describes my own personal and professional journey. In this book, I detail my voyage from a middle-class American child curious about God, science, ESP, and the mind, through what I now see as a necessary detour as a corporate technology strategist, to my current role as a psychotherapist, with a clinical philosophy inspired and informed by psychedelic drugs.

Today, Harvard, Johns Hopkins, New York University, the University of California—Los Angeles, and a few other of the most prestigious medical schools worldwide are conducting clinical research with psychedelics in a psychiatric context. Studies are once again under way to assess the utility of psychedelic chemicals to ease anxiety in the dying, to interrupt the hold of addictive drugs, and to cure post-traumatic stress disorder and other deeply felt, heartbreaking conditions. While psychedelic substances are not a panacea—there are no magic bullets—results to date have been very positive, and psychedelics, when used carefully in a professional context, are now being accepted by the medical community as a powerful psychiatric—and spiritual—medicine.

I use the term *spiritual medicine* specifically, because it is becoming clear that the curative effect of psychedelic drugs comes not from triggering a mechanical effect in the body, but rather by engendering a peak or spiritual experience. (Even subjects who are atheists have a profound sense of the wholeness of the universe and their place within it.) This finding—that the desired clinical effect comes through a "spiritual" experience—is changing the very definition of what it means to be a psychiatrist, of the field of medicine, and of modern society at the most fundamental of levels.

For me, the challenge in writing this book was to communicate this area of medical research and professional clinical practice that until recently has been hidden from even the educated, intelligent public, while using my own journey to impart my deeply felt personal and professional growth experience—and finally to assist and give root to my own on–going process of discovery and maturation. Of course, every author faces the personal challenge of transforming a blank page to a volume such as the one you now hold in your hands, and every volume is a statement of the author's values. I have built this book, this exercise in reviewing—seeing something new—on a foundation of research and scholarship going back millennia, particularly on that period of increasing research and scholarship spanning the past 125 years. I offer my sincerest appreciation to my entire reference list for providing me with a rich field of ideas to re-see, and I take sole responsibility for all my statements in this book, including any errors.

Introduction

THE QUESTIONS THAT LED TO THIS BOOK

As I have pursued my exploration of psychedelics and personal change, and as I've developed my own clinical practice, I have challenged myself to keep a focus on the effectiveness of psychotherapy and of psychedelics for personality development, change, and transformation. After all, if psychotherapy and psychedelics don't work "as advertised," we're at best wasting time and at worst challenging ourselves unnecessarily, personally, professionally, and societally. What follows then are the questions I've asked myself—ultimately, the questions I have been called upon to address in this book.

The first and foremost question I want to explore is: Can psychedelics be a distraction from personal development? In a world short on miracles and grace, the field of psychedelics makes many seemingly magical claims. To name just a few of the many hopes and expectations of the psychedelic community, it has been claimed that psychedelics can:

- ► cure alcoholism
- ► turn off a "switch" in the brain to alleviate opiate addiction
- ► restore empathy in couples
- ► provide transformative change in psychotherapy
- ► enable one to see God (and talk with her!)
- ► bestow enlightenment

1

In Western culture, it is a given that spiritual maturity is associated with years of meditation or study, yet psychedelics hold the promise of "enlightenment in a pill." Might I and others of my generation have been seduced by the easy mysticism offered by psychedelics, perhaps expecting one-shot bliss and so being dissuaded from the rigors of non-drug-related therapies or spiritual practices (practices that ironically may be necessary to sustain and integrate psychedelic insights)?

Individuals can try to avoid the arduous process of building wisdom by expecting psychedelics to simply transform them. In the youth world of the psychedelic '60s, there tended to be a cynicism toward the hierarchical, organized gathering of knowledge along with a bias toward direct, primary experience unprocessed by analysis, rather than a desire for balance between the two.

These attitudes prevailed in the '60s mostly because the potential risks of psychedelics were generally unknown, or, if known, generally flaunted. Though the attitudes of the '60s are not the same today, the question still remains as to whether psychedelics are a benefit to personal development or a distraction. Though I will show throughout the course of this book that I believe they hold great promise, the contraindications and risks are real and need to be considered for each individual in making the choice to use them. The first and foremost risk to be aware of revolves around a personal or family history of mental illness with psychotic or schizoid elements. For the genetically predisposed, psychedelics could trigger the onset of symptoms.

In addition to psychotic susceptibility in those with family predisposition, one of the more important concerns about the safety of using these substances for personal development is the question of whether or not psychedelics might be associated with or could cause developmental impairment. The most important predictors of developmental impairment associated with the use of psychedelics are age and frequency of use—the younger the user and the more frequent the use, the greater the likelihood of developmental impairment, social and/or cognitive.

Young, frequent users' susceptibility to developmental impairment brings me to my most important contraindication: immaturity. In fact, I used to joke during talks that "no one under forty should be allowed to take psychedelics." After the good-natured jeers had stopped and the audience had settled back down, we would discuss how the audience feels about restricting the use of psychedelics to an older cohort and why I might have made that provocative statement. In fact, I don't believe it to be true, since the most frequent integration of psychedelics into common tribal use is around times of change and rites of passage, including the transformation from child to teen and from teen to adult. I am ultimately making a point about the importance of mind-set, receptivity, and preparedness—that is, mature intentionality—for the effective use of psychedelics. Unfortunately, in the West, our children encounter these powerful substances without the support and guidance of experienced elders. In cases of developmental impairment in youths, the problem is also correlated with the quality of the home environment and in particular the quality of parenting.

So, with the above caveats in mind, the question still remains: Is psychedelic therapy a useful tool for lasting change in adults? Over the course of this book, I specifically want to explore the following questions:

- Can psychedelic therapy repair malfunctions in natural development?
- Can psychedelic therapy speed up the natural developmental process?
- Can psychedelic therapy trigger immediate transformative change in novel areas?

In trying to answer these questions, I will discuss the exciting new clinical research that reconsiders the original role of psychedelic chemicals as spectacularly powerful psychiatric medicines. Most people have not heard of this particular line of research; this is where my interest in research coincides with my interest in things *crypto-*, or "hidden."

Psychedelic plants have been well integrated into tribal societies globally for millennia, yet Western civilization fights them. What is the hidden history of psychedelics in society, in medicine, and religion? Now that psychedelic therapy research is under way again at prestigious medical schools worldwide, will the new research be shut down, as it was the last time? Or will a more accepting, post-1960s generation of decision makers permit the research to continue, ultimately building a new psychiatry?

This brings me to the next set of questions I address in the book. If this research is indeed allowed to continue, as I hope it will, investigators will need to address several thorny theoretical and methodological questions:

- ▶ Why does psychedelic research require self-experimentation and, because of this need, how will we train a new generation of psychedelic researchers and therapists?
- ▶ Why redo psychedelic research already conducted in the '50s and '60s?
- ▶ How should psychedelics be rescheduled?
- ▶ How regulated should the use of psychedelics become?
- ▶ Why do psychedelics give pain relief?
- ▶ Can psychedelics provide lasting change?
- ▶ Can psychedelics induce real spirituality, and are they a medicine or a sacrament?

Assuming these questions can be resolved, and I believe many already have, the next question becomes:

- ▶ Will the results of the current spate of medical school–based clinical research with patients be positive enough to justify acceptance of psychedelics as having an official medical use?

The last question that I'll address on the clinical use of psychedelics will be:

▸ If the results are positive and the outstanding issues are addressed, how will psychedelics be integrated into medicine, science, and society—and how might that change the world?

In addition to discussing the clinical research literature on psychedelics, I will also explore a new approach to clinical psychology, one that is based on development rather than on pathology, one that focuses on love and the soul rather than on using pharmaceuticals as the weapon of first choice. I call this new approach "psycheology" to remind us that the term *psychology* was built on the root word *psyche* (Greek for "soul") and so should again become the study of our core self, not the medical approach to controlling the mind with pharmaceuticals into which it has devolved.

While we're asking clinical questions, let's ask what exactly is personality—and is personality the true, basic self? Does psychotherapy actually change people? As asked above, what is the role of psychedelics in psychological development and psychotherapy? What is the psycheology model of developmental change? How does this all apply at the societal level?

In our approach to personal development, we must understand both the term *development* and the underlying concept of change. But what do we mean by *change*? Do we mean growth, as in adding more? Do we mean maturation, in the sense of growing older and more capable? Do we mean development that goes through a series of stages? What about transformation—what is it that would be transformed, into what, and by what process? It's even more important to ask: Is change even the right goal for psychotherapy? Might acceptance be a more appropriate goal?

Since I don't believe in a medical approach to what I view as essentially a *developmental* process, one of the primary questions this book addresses is if personality change is possible and desirable, and how change can best be brought about, if not through the traditional clinical approach.

To answer this question, we'll begin at the beginning, by exploring the concept of change at its most fundamental level—starting in math and physics. We'll continue to explore and define change in biology and human development, and ultimately focus on the meaning and process of change on the societal and spiritual levels (even for nonspiritual readers).

This book will also detail the psycheology perspective—the origins of psychology as the study of the psyche, or soul—to understanding the process of personality development and maturation, and will describe the practice of psychotherapy based on the clinical philosophy of psychology. Finally, this book will describe the longer-term implications of the psychology worldview for an integral society—one that integrates the mature use of psychedelics into the process of change, growth, and maturation, on the individual and the societal levels.

But first, let us begin by exploring how a middle-aged, middle-class psychologist came to be taking a psychedelic drug, alone in his apartment, surrounded by Post-it Notes.

I

SET AND SETTING

THE MOTHER OF ALL TRIPS

My purpose in taking "acid"—in 1991, eighteen years after my use of psychedelics in college—was to see if, after all those years, I had sold out my youthful ideals, if I had slowly, imperceptibly, become a person I could no longer respect. My goal was to lift up and look at the root ball of my life's plant, but not to undertake a complete transplant—and I was terrified of what I might find.

I chose a day when I could be alone in my apartment. Although I did have friends on call, I wanted to have this experience on my own. Anticipating something similar to what I had experienced in my college days in the 1960s, I pulled out my old psychedelic music albums—*The Jimi Hendrix Experience,* the Beatles' *Sgt. Pepper's Lonely Hearts Club Band,* and the like. Since I was so scared of the experience—might I go screaming down the street, pulling my hair out, and end up in a mental hospital?—I decided to place Post-it Notes around the apartment with reassuring phrases such as "Don't worry; it's only a drug" and "You'll be down soon." I then swallowed half a square blotter paper dose and waited.

I knew from my research that contemporary doses of LSD were nowhere near the strength of what I'd experienced in the '60s—the average dose was a modest 80 micrograms or so, compared with the clinical dose of 150 micrograms, the purported dose of 250 micrograms in the famed "orange sunshine" tabs, and the whopping 450 micrograms sometimes necessary in psychedelic therapy with alcoholics. When the acid began to come on, I felt a very minor fluttering in my belly, some slight increase in color, and some waviness in the lights and then . . . nothing. It all faded away. I thought, "After all this preparation, I got a weak disco dose," and I took the other half of the blotter. A few minutes later, the first half started to come on in full force.

Of course, I'd forgotten one of the first rules of tripping that I'd learned in the '60s: psychedelics come on in waves. The first wave tends to be just noticeable, often in a slight feeling in the belly. This first wave frequently subsides below the noticeable level, but is soon followed by subsequent waves that get stronger. I immediately remembered why I had taken these substances so seriously in my youth and realized I was in for a stronger ride than I'd planned.

Traveler's Guide

Here are some other rules I wrote down around that time.

Things to bring along when traveling:

▶ music (happy, positive, serene)

▶ fresh flowers and fruit

▶ art books

▶ yoga music

Things to remember when traveling:

▶ "Turn off your mind, relax and float downstream; it is not dying, it is not dying. Lay down all thoughts, surrender to the void; it is shining, it is shining. That you may know the meaning of within; it is being, it is being." —John Lennon, "Tomorrow Never Knows," *Revolver,* January 1966, closely adapted from *The Psychedelic Experience: A Manual Based on the Tibetan Book of the Dead,* by Timothy Leary, Ralph Metzner, and Richard Alpert, which in turn was adapted from the *Tibetan Book of the Dead.*

▶ "Sit down, shut up, and pay attention." —Terence McKenna

▶ Surrender.

▶ Ask "What am I feeling?"

Broadly speaking, there are four stages to the psychedelic experience:

▶ Sensory/visual—including generally pleasant visual distortions and amplification, appreciation for sounds and music, enhanced pleasure in physical touch, and so forth.

▶ Psychological/recollecto/analytical—subconscious work on childhood issues, emotions, and the like.

▶ Holistic/ecological/mythic—history of the species and of the planet, the march of evolution, sense of the global whole.

▶ Integral/white light/ego death—dissociation from personal, individual identity and physical existence, replaced by identity with universal energy.

> —Adapted from R. E. L. Masters, Ph.D., and Jean Houston, Ph.D., *The Varieties of Psychedelic Experience,* 1966

More things to remember when traveling:

▶ Don't forget the fruit and the water.

▶ Caffeine is a two-edged sword. It increases attention, but cushions against emotions. Best to avoid except perhaps toward the end as a refresher.

▶ Marijuana can enhance, sustain, and rejuvenate the experience but not really increase the effect.

▶ Writing is a two-edged sword. It captures the experience, but focuses attention through one medium. Best to avoid using a computer throughout; maybe keep a pad and pen around to capture important epiphanies. That being said, the truly important insights are memorable.

▶ After an often uncertain first hour or two, the longer, remaining part of the trip can be a beautiful, benevolent, natural, wondrous experience.

▶ Don't be macho'd into taking megadoses. More may be

appropriate for certain fields of study, but for psychological purposes, just significantly noticeable can be very effective. At lower levels, sensory experiences can be ignored and yet significant benefits can result.

► Don't think you are down enough to answer the phone. It will be your mother-in-law. There is a law of the universe that states that specifically. Even if it's not, the conversation will more often than not be stressful for one or both of you.

► To maximize psychological growth, don't get distracted by the pretty, dancing visuals. Breathe and go deeper.

Tripping has sometimes been compared to a roller-coaster ride: at first, the car goes up and up and up, with the feeling that the climbing will never end and we will go up forever, never to come down. Like a roller coaster, however, once the trip reaches its peak, despite many dramatic ups and downs, the ascent is over. On my "mother of all trips," once I felt the upward trajectory ease, I knew I would not "go through the roof" and began to feel safe and relaxed.

It was at this point that I had a profound internal experience, what I think of as a waking dream or eyes-closed vision: I was in a beautiful valley field of purple flowers with surrounding mountains in the background. As I continued to come on to the experience, I found myself descending deeper and deeper, eventually going below the surface of the ground (I generally don't think of such experiences as going "higher"; rather, I feel that I am going down, into my deeper self). At that point, I saw the roots of the flowers—they looked animal-like, not like plant roots, but more like the thick tails of hairless moles—and in this dreamlike vision, I knew that they were my (psychological) roots. As I had just begun my trip and so still retained much of my "straight"-mind, operant perspective, I decided to examine them and fix any problems, so I visually zoomed in for a better look. As soon as I approached with this proactive, problem-solving attitude, my roots recoiled from my scrutiny, curling back and emitting a high-pitched, scared squeal. This response made me feel uneasy, and to avoid a vicious cycle of negativity, I mentally and visually turned the other direction and continued my descent. As I did and moved deeper, I saw at the bottom of me, a glowing, throbbing orb, that I knew was "the ground of my being." As I descended and reached the orb, I touched it and immediately felt at peace. I finally remembered the important truths—that I was essentially OK, that love and acceptance were the fundamental solutions to my problems, in fact, that the "problems" I was grappling with were really just poignant developmental challenges, that I had not "sold out my youthful ideals" or become someone I couldn't respect, and that my only problem was my sense that I had problems.

At that point, I began to ascend, back up from my depths toward the surface, where I saw my roots again. This time, however, instead of wanting to fix my roots, I felt enormous compassion and total acceptance. This time, I reached out to caress my roots with the attitude, "Of course. I understand. It's OK." In response, my roots unfurled, opening to my touch, and emitted a low-pitched sigh of safety, peace, and relaxation.

The experience was transformative in many ways—providing me with a clear understanding of our essential OK-ness as well as inspiring the personality theory underlying my soon-to-be-reestablished clinical practice.

Here is a poem I wrote about that experience:

Missed, Mist

I feel in a mist
Sleepwalking through life
Sleeptalking with other sleepwalkers
Triggering out my insides

On the other hand . . .

I float down to my ground

And on the way down
I cry my childhood into completion
On the ground
A glowing mound throbs,
Emanating peace

I touch the glowing orb
And my sleeping seed awakens
Reigniting the unfolding frozen so long ago
Unfolding unto the sun
Upward to the warmth of love
From the glow to the warmth

My worldview changed from an evaluation-analysis-repair-of-pathology model to one of essential all-rightness and acceptance, of maturation and spiritual development. Through that one experience, I came to see that we are, in essence, perfect at our core—and that insight informed my sense of myself and my approach to my clinical practice:

- ▶ Psychology is the study of the psyche, the soul—the ground of our being;
- ▶ Personality is acquired, secondary, external, defensive, strategic—a shell above our core of fundamental perfection; and
- ▶ Love, empathy, and compassion form a more effective perspective for healthy, satisfying personal development than does the medical "fix-it" approach focused on pathology.

WHO I AM

Since this is such a personal book and one with a unique premise, it's important for you, the reader, to know who I am, where I've come from, and what my credentials are to make such demands on your worldview.

My background includes both psychotherapy and policy research, and today I am both a psychotherapist in private practice and a drug policy analyst and writer. I am an expert in the clinical use of psychedelics, yet I don't use them in my practice. Why not? Two reasons. First, they are illegal, and I would be putting much of my life at risk if I were to use them with clients. (Not *patients*. Remember, I take a developmental, not a pathology, approach to my clinical practice.) Second, I am not qualified to do psychedelic therapy—and almost no one is, simply because there is still no legal way to conduct psychedelic therapy outside the auspices of an approved research project, so the career path for a psychedelic psychotherapist is at the moment quite limited. And there are no clinical training programs in psychedelic therapy. That may change over the next five years or so, but for now a psychotherapist with a private practice in psychedelic psychotherapy does so illegally and almost certainly without clinical training.* Even those therapists who do have training and experience with psychedelics gained when they were legal have no legal way to practice in this area.

So I remain a scholar of psychedelic therapy, but not a psychedelic therapist, except in very important sense that my experiences with psychedelics have fundamentally shaped my clinical practice.

One way to describe my background is to tell you about my experience at the local middle school's Career Day. Yes, despite my specialty in psychedelics (they probably didn't Google me), I have three times been invited to speak to local middle-school kids on what it's like to be a psychologist. In preparing for such a lovely and important responsibility, I reviewed my background and can confidently say that I am a poster child for the range and diversity of the field of psychology. As I told the kids, I have been a counselor and group therapist; a policy researcher

---

*William (Bill) A. Richards, Ph.D., a psychologist and lead psychedelic guide on the current Johns Hopkins Psilocybin Cancer Project, also conducted psychedelic therapy research at the Maryland Psychiatric Research Center in the early 1970s and, before that, at Harvard in the early 1960s. Richards has worked with psychedelics throughout his thoughtful, soulful career and is a treasured resource of hard-won knowledge, experience, and wisdom for the psychedelic therapy and research community. More on Richards later.

specializing in the utilization of new research; an internal consultant on innovation and change; a corporate strategic planner focused on the use of advanced technology; a publisher and editor of paper and online publications on organizational development and change management; a professor of business strategy and policy; a conference planner, speaker curator, and master of ceremonies; a public speaker; a published writer in the scholarly literature, and now in books; and since 2001, a psychotherapist—all quite comfortably fitting under the professional umbrella of the field of psychology. If you are interested in a career in psychology, you certainly need not feel hemmed in by the image of a psychologist as a clinician!

But how did this poster boy for professional psychology come to be swallowing LSD at the ripe old age of forty-one?

HOW I BECAME INTERESTED IN CONSCIOUSNESS AND PSYCHEDELIC THERAPY

As far back as I can remember, I was the bookish type and always interested in the unusual, the anomalous, the exception that *dis*proves the rule, paradigm shifts, quantum jumps, the corners of the envelope, and beyond. As a child, I was fascinated by questions of immortality and the existence of God. One of my first mind twisters was a kind of Western koan that went around in the late 1950s: "What happens when an irresistible force meets an immovable object?" Later on, in the mid-1960s, in junior high school and high school, I remember admiring Gandhi's impossible-yet-successful civil disobedience and pondering Einstein's concept of the universe as boundless yet finite. I told our rabbi that if he owned more than one suit, he was a hypocrite, and I was intrigued by Eastern philosophy, as well as by Bob Dylan's and the Beatles' use of LSD (as described in *Time* magazine, which my parents received)—although I was much too scared to try it, unlike some of my junior high school friends, who took sugar cubes of LSD (in school!) before it was made illegal in October of 1968.

Later, I took an interest in Charles Fort's compilations of ephemeral facts, and later still, in a more sophisticated version of Fort's work, William Corliss's Sourcebook Project* on anomalous mental or natural phenomena. Both Fort and especially Corliss collect documentable examples of phenomena that are true but rare and thus frequently dismissed as impossible. Logic and rationality should prevail, even when the phenomenon is unusual. Even to this day, my salon Poetry Science Talks (www.poetrysciencetalks.com) focuses on unusual topics, and one of my favorite books is *The Future of the Body: Explorations into the Further Evolution of Human Nature,* by Esalen Institute cofounder Michael Murphy, which provides an encyclopedic overview of the multitude of techniques employed over the centuries to speed human development.[1] With this history, it should be no surprise that I pursued a doctorate in psychology and have an interest in psychedelics.

I have always focused on being part of a larger society and on being helpful. When I was a college sophomore I participated in a professor's research study, ostensibly about visual pattern recognition, but in reality about the ethics of helping behavior. After sitting in the dark, drawing a lightbulb's apparent motion,[†] I was brought into the professor's office to be debriefed. While I was sitting there, the next subject came to the door and apologized for not being able to participate in the study as scheduled. "Why not?" asked the professor. "Actually, I'm tripping on LSD and having a bad time." Then the student said, "Can you tell me where I can get some help?" "No, I'm afraid not," replied the professor. Concerned, I craned my neck to see the student (he was holding back a bit, so I had to actively move to see him), and I told him that the nearby Free Clinic could help him. When he didn't respond, I asked if he knew where the

---

*For example see: W. R. Corliss, *The Unfathomed Mind: A Handbook of Unusual Mental Phenomena* (Glen Arm, Md.: Sourcebook Project, 1982); or W. R. Corliss, *Handbook of Unusual Natural Phenomena* (Glen Arm, Md.: Sourcebook Project, 1977).

†The retina will soon adapt to a point of light that will soon seem to disappear. To avoid this, the eye continually moves slightly so as to expose different rod cells to the stimuli, thus making sure the light source remains seen. The side effect is that the light will appear to move around—apparent motion.

free clinic was. "Uh . . . no," was his response. "OK," I said. "We're almost done here. Why don't I take you over?" The student looked at the professor, and the professor looked at the student and then back at me. It turned out that the student was actually a confederate of the researcher and that this exchange comprised the real study—which was of altruistic behavior. The professor told me that most subjects lean back to avoid the "student" and that it was unusual for the subject to offer to actually walk with the student to get help. I attribute my response to being part of a subculture where such behavior was the norm.

My interest in applied research and impact on policy began when I took twin courses in my senior year of college at Case-Western Reserve University: Seminar and Practicum in Adult Psychopathology and Seminar and Practicum in Child Psychopathology. The course in adult psychopathology took place in an actual lunatic asylum. Built in the 1870s as the Northern Ohio Lunatic Asylum and later renamed the Cleveland State Hospital, this facility was black, turreted, and fortress-like. Subjected to budget cuts during the deinstitutionalization movement of the 1960s and '70s, the institution featured bare lightbulbs; bare walls that curved right into the ceilings (thus creating an amplifying, reverberating, hallucinogenic effect on all noise); and the constant sounds of moaning, crying, and bizarre singing of the psychotic residents (off-key, a cappella renditions of "Over the Rainbow" would be a typical undertone). If one were not insane upon arrival, this facility could have easily accomplished the task. I quickly realized that no effective psychotherapy could be conducted there. The physical environment and the state's public policy were having the greatest impact on the mental health of its residents (staff included!), rather than any attempts at individual psychological treatment. I certainly had little impact on the psychotic resident I was assigned to talk with.

By contrast, my child seminar and practicum took place at Sagamore Hills Children Psychiatric Hospital, in Northfield, Ohio, the state's showpiece. Although at the time (1973) Ohio was second to last (after Alabama) in state funding for mental health services, Sagamore Hills was well funded. There were social workers galore, a great teacher-to-student ratio, and sophisticated teaching technologies, such as computers that could ask questions and provide rewards for correct answers. In addition, carpeting, beautiful wall art, and lounge areas abounded. All the staff worked together under the rubric of "milieu therapy," in which everyone from janitors to kitchen staff to administrative directors considered it part of their job to contribute to patient outcome. Sporting pastel walls, ample sunlight, and tree-lined walks, this facility seemed to heal kids through its positive environment alone.

After taking these two courses, it became obvious that the institutional environment and the mental health policy underlying that environment have a powerful yet subtle and often underappreciated impact on patient outcome.

After graduating from Case-Western with a bachelor's degree in psychology and a 4.0 grade point average my last three semesters, I entered the master's program in counselor education at New York University (NYU). I received my master's degree in counseling from NYU, with training in occupational and educational counseling and specialization in psychological counseling. I did my internship at the Central Counseling Service, under the late Reverend Theodore R. Smith Jr., a Unitarian Universalist minister specializing in chaplaincy and pastoral counseling. I worked with Ted because he was the best role model for a spiritual approach to personal development.

Upon receiving my master's degree, I realized that I was more interested in and better suited to a research focus. Although I had always been intrigued by the far corners of science and the mind—God, ESP, cosmology, and the like—I have always had a coincident interest in fact-based decision making and a desire to have an impact on the world. I viewed (and still view) pure, speculative thought as an indulgence, unless it is based on research—the "best of what is known"—and wedded to impact, applying what we know toward improving the real world. I remember the turning point in this decision process came in one of Ted's therapy groups, in which I was affectionately referred to as the T.I.T.—therapist in training. One woman was having a weight problem—she complained to the group that "every time I see the refrigerator, I just can't help but open it up and eat something." My response—thankfully kept to myself—was, "Just don't do that—you're fat!" At that point, I knew it was either found a new school of thought called Kick-in-the-Ass therapy, or put my counseling career on hold and pursue my interest in research.

While my academic momentum propelled me to get my master's in a clinical discipline, counseling, it eventually became apparent that if I wanted to have the greatest impact on the suffering and the mental health of patients, I would have to focus my training not on one-to-one clinical psychology, not on group psychotherapy, not even on directing a mental health facility, but on policy research. In order to have the strongest patient impact, I needed to concentrate on the factors that facilitate or inhibit research-based change in mental health policy.

In 1976, I decided to pursue a doctorate in applied research and action science,* and I entered the public affairs psychology program in social/environmental psychology at Claremont Graduate School (now the Claremont Graduate University) in Claremont, California.

The Claremont colleges (Pomona, Scripps, Claremont McKenna, Harvey Mudd, Pitzer, and the Claremont Graduate University) are each oriented toward public service. In the graduate social/environmental psychology program at Claremont, that means training students to conduct research, not in a laboratory with two-way mirrors, with white rats (or graduate students) as subjects, but rather in the field—on street corners, in schools, in mental hospitals, and in community mental health centers. This format is similar to sociology, but with the methodological rigor traditionally associated with lab psychology.

The public affairs psychology program was the "baby" of Arthur H. Brayfield, a former executive officer of the American Psychological

---

*Action science is an approach to research that focuses on generating knowledge that is useful in solving practical problems (from http://en.wikipedia.org/wiki/Chris_Argyris).

Association and, despite his advancing age and white hair, an unregenerate "hippie" who had brought his humanistic social consciousness to bear in the founding of the program. In practical terms, this meant training students to become program evaluation researchers, with graduate students typically taking jobs in schools or mental health facilities doing internal research to assess the efficacy of various educational or psychological programs.

Given my focus on having an impact on policy and society, it should come as no surprise that I became interested in the utility of the evaluation research reports we were being trained to conduct. In fact, it was in Art Brayfield's first-year research methods class that I first broached the question of how all these evaluation research reports were being used, and was—quickly and quietly, it now occurs to me—handed a copy of Ronald G. Havelock's book *Planning for Innovation through Dissemination and Utilization of Knowledge*. It was as close as I've ever come to a "the scales fell from my eyes" experience. While my specialization at Claremont was officially in applied research methods, this was the beginning of my interest in policy research utilization, ultimately the topic of my dissertation.

Ron Havelock was then at the Center for Research on Utilization of Scientific Knowledge, at the Institute for Social Research at the University of Michigan in Ann Arbor (and was later to become one of my many mentors in the field). As I read in this area, I became more enamored with its logic: the failure to use valid and reliable policy research is worse than worthless; it is a staggeringly huge opportunity cost, a waste of resources that might have been applied elsewhere. Of course, the more I focused not on evaluation research, but on the meta issue of its use, the less my Claremont faculty was interested in my meta research focus. To most of them, "good research will, perforce, be implemented, given enough time." Yet time is exactly what we don't have: time to waste conducting research in a way that would never be implemented into policy nor deployed into practice.

If studying hospitals could have more impact than conducting psychotherapy on individual and small groups, and if studying mental health policy could have more impact than studying individual hospitals, then studying the utilization of mental health policy research—assuring that mental health policy and practice is based on state-of-the-art research—could have the greatest impact of all. I was in love with that topic, but unfortunately without a thesis advisor—none of my faculty was interested in a field that could call into question the raison d'être of their entire academic lives. Once I passed my oral qualifying exams and was ready to begin my dissertation research, after a systematic search process, I found a research position working under one of the "fathers of the field," Robert F. Rich, a political science professor at the Woodrow Wilson School of Public and International Affairs at Princeton University. I was ready to move back East.

I worked for Bob Rich as deputy principal investigator of a three-year, federally funded study focusing precisely on mental health policy research utilization. I supervised the staff of undergraduate research assistants; juggled the budget; conducted interviews with directors of mental health facilities and regulatory bodies at the local, state, and federal levels; analyzed our questionnaire data using the nonparametric statistics I'd just learned at Claremont; reported on our progress to our funding agency, the National Institute of Mental Health (NIMH); and co-wrote papers with Bob that were published in scholarly journals. Most important, I was able to use our data to write my doctoral dissertation. I was one fortunate graduate student!

In addition to our NIMH grant to study mental health policy research utilization, we also had a special National Science Foundation grant to help develop the fledgling academic field of research utilization. Part of that grant was meant to support communication among the researchers in the field, and toward that end, we convened small invited conferences, bringing in all the key researchers in the field, such as University of Michigan psychologist Ron Havelock, Harvard sociologist Carol H. Weiss, and psychologists Edward Glaser and Thomas Backer of the Human Interaction Research Institute in California. I was the one responsible for organizing and administering these small meetings of the leading researchers in the field, including getting them from the Princeton Junction train station to their hotel rooms! In the process, I got to sit at the feet of my idols—the scholars I had been citing in my term papers back at Claremont—and gained valuable, on-the-ground experience in bringing together leading thinkers for purposes of knowledge transfer and dissemination. This is one of the surest ways to push forward any field of endeavor and facilitate change in policy, practice, and society. This skill—"the care and feeding of gurus"—was to become a major and continuing thread in my career.

After my mentor Bob Rich lost a messy fight for tenure at Princeton, I left academia, feeling bruised and sullied. My attitude at the time, rightly or wrongly, was "If I'm going to have to deal with this sort of jealousy, bickering, and competitiveness, I might as well be paid for it." After one more year with Bob Rich at The School of Urban and Public Affairs at Carnegie Mellon University, I took a position as a research associate in the Technology and Productivity (TaP) Research Center at AT&T in Piscataway, New Jersey.

My new manager, Rob Epstein, was familiar with the research utilization field and on hiring me he told me, "You know that research utilization field you've been studying? Well, we do the same thing here, except it's research-based *technology* you'll be utilizing—I want you to do the same thing within AT&T in the form of technology transfer and implementation." It turned out that the two fields were remarkably similar. Valid and reliable research-based technology is often not adopted, due to a range of factors, such as the famous "not-invented-here" syndrome, wherein members of an organization reject perfectly valid recommendations simply because they come from the outside, are unfamiliar, and will require the admission of ignorance and the climbing of an at-times steep learning curve.

In my job at TaP, I was an internal consultant for planned organizational change, assessing the level of readiness for innovative technology, introducing new tools based on artificial intelligence (AI), and measuring progress as the organization incorporated—or rejected—the new technology. We had many successes and quite a few informative failures in bringing AI technology into use within AT&T. I also worked with Bell Labs to develop new AI-based products. And as at Princeton, I was also responsible for convening small gatherings of vendors and researchers working at the state-of-the-art in this emerging area, to disseminate this knowledge within AT&T. I should point out that when I arrived at AT&T, I knew literally nothing about artificial intelligence, but by the time I left, I had become quite expert in this new field, in particular on how to assess organizational need for the technology and which applications would be most useful given the organization's mission. I also became very knowledgeable about the products and fledgling companies developing new AI hardware and software products to address corporate needs. It was based on this new expertise that I took my next job, as a research analyst covering the marketplace for AI technologies at an information technology market research and consulting firm, Gartner Group (now simply Gartner, Inc.).

At Gartner, I covered the marketplace for artificial intelligence, creating research reports assessing innovations in artificial intelligence; speaking at Gartner conferences; and consulting with clients on their best path for evaluating, selecting, and implementing artificial intelligence tools. Gartner was a very commercial and competitive environment, and eventually I left, taking my dream job as director of technology strategy in the strategic planning department of American Express Company, in the corporate headquarters located in the World Financial Center, right across the street from the World Trade Towers in lower Manhattan.

I call the Amex position my dream job because it was everything I had been striving toward in corporate America. It was a research job focused on the future. It was in the strategic planning department, and my boss reported to the chairman of the company. I had a multimillion-dollar budget for emerging technology research and was responsible for deciding which projects would be conducted by the advanced technology groups in each of our six subsidiaries. I conducted internal consulting engagements to facilitate the diffusion and deployment of the latest emerging technology across the company. My office was on the forty-fifth floor of the World Financial Center with a stunning view of the Manhattan skyline—with the Empire State Building, the Chrysler Building, and the Hudson River sparkling before me. Also, as had become the norm in my career, I was responsible for convened gatherings—both online and for the chairman and the board of directors—of the most innovative small vendors and most knowledgeable gurus in the fields of artificial intelligence, the World Wide Web (which had just been invented by Tim Berners-Lee and Robert Cailliau), research-based technology transfer, and organizational innovation and change. To me, this was the best job in corporate America: it utilized my unique constellation of skills perfectly, it enabled me to study change and apply it in real-world settings in ways that had concrete impact, and I was paid obscenely well.

And I was miserable.

Was I dissatisfied because I had just turned forty—an age I'd always thought of deep inside as the time by which I'd have hung out a shingle and started a private practice? Was it because I felt completely alienated from the typical sales-and-marketing-oriented executive at American Express? Was it because I had come to realize that even in my "sexy" emerging technology strategy job, I was really just using artificial intelligence and the Internet—that my mind and soul were being used—to help American Express pick our pockets ever more effectively? Of course, it was because of all of these reasons, but the central, primary catalyst for my dissatisfaction was the fact that, after a hiatus of almost twenty years, I had quietly begun taking psychedelics again. I was ready for—crying out for—a more meaningful, more human-scale life, and psychedelics provided the lever out.

HOW I GOT TO BE WHO I AM NOW

It was actually a close relative who told me about MDMA (the drug known as Ecstasy). She explained what it was and suggested that I do it with my wife. At this point in my life, I hadn't done any psychedelics for almost twenty years.

Back in college I did my tripping (maybe twenty-five to fifty trips; mostly lysergic acid diethylamide-25, or LSD) without the benefit of reading any of the research. In fact, although I was a psychology major and (I later learned) there were thousands of peer-reviewed research papers in the literature, none of the clinical research was ever mentioned in any of my courses or textbooks. Of course, there were the obligatory warnings about the Russian roulette possibility of psychotic reactions to "hallucinogens,"* but nothing about the tantalizingly suggestive findings from the clinical research pointing to the potential to help the dying or to treat alcoholism, to name just two of the many applications being studied at the time.† (I say "suggestive" research findings because despite the many peer-reviewed journal articles on the clinical research with psychedelics conducted between the late 1940s and the early 1970s, there were still no large-scale, epidemiological research studies to

---

*In this book, I will use the word *hallucinogen* in discussing the medical research and the word *psychedelic* in most other contexts. The words refer to the same drugs, but in differing contexts (and so to different experiences). The word *hallucinogen* is actually a misnomer, as the "classic hallucinogens"—mescaline, LSD, psilocybin—rarely produce sensory experiences that have no basis in reality, e.g., seeing and talking with a person who is not really present. Rather, the hallucinogens are most likely to produce visual distortions of sensory input that is actually present, e.g., seeing actual lights as spreading out or trailing behind the source, or seeing flat surfaces such as walls or floors as seeming to breathe or undulate. Plants in the Solanaceae (nightshades) family contain scopolamine, atropine, and hyoscyamine, the active ingredients in the herbalist "witches" hexing herbs. These chemicals can produce true hallucinations, such as the illusion of talking to the devil, but these deliriants are definitely not psychedelic in the soul-manifesting way in which we are approaching them in this book.

†Other application areas researched have included: creativity; criminal recidivism (?)— the question mark reflects the flawed methodology of the research that attempted to demonstrate this application; cluster headaches; substance abuse and addiction, especially alcoholism; relationship counseling; childhood autism; post-traumatic stress disorder; depression; obsessive-compulsive disorder; pain relief; end-stage psychotherapy with the dying (mostly cancer and more recently AIDS); facilitation of the meditative state; and elicitation of mystical experience. I will discuss most of these in as we review the history of psychedelic research in chapter 3.

validate the positive results found in many of those initial studies. Even now, during the current renaissance in psychedelic research, there still have been no such large-sample studies conducted to follow up on any of those promising—tantalizing—early studies.)

~~~

Throughout my rediscovery and exploration of psychedelics, I was fortunate to be guided by many brilliant, generous mentors. These profiles highlight some—but not all—of these extraordinary luminaries.

Profile: David Lukoff, Ph.D.

One of the first individuals I was fortunate to encounter was professor David G. Lukoff of the Saybrook Graduate School in San Francisco. Dr. Lukoff is a licensed psychologist whose areas of expertise include the treatment of schizophrenia, transpersonal psychology, spiritual issues in clinical practice, and case study methodology. He is co-author of the "Religious or Spiritual Problems" diagnostic category for the *Diagnostic and Statistical Manual of Mental Disorders,* fourth edition (DSM-IV). Dr. Lukoff had co-written an influential paper discussing the mostly ethnographic research on psychedelics that had still been possible during the "big freeze" between the late 1970s and the early 1990s; and in 1991, I called him to ask for some professional guidance.[2] During that conversation, as I outlined my background in policy research utilization, he said, "Hmm. That sounds incredibly relevant to psychedelics." I was confused and asked him what he meant. He replied, "Well, you're trained in research utilization, and psychedelic research is perhaps the most-underutilized valid and reliable research there is." Amazingly, that connection hadn't yet occurred to me, but of course it was true. Due to the controversial, challenging nature of psychedelic phenomena, valid and reliable psychedelic research had long been underadopted into policy—and so, underutilized in clinical practice. Encouraged by Dr. Lukoff, I resolved to make use of my expertise in research utilization to assist in the creation and use of valid and reliable research about psychedelics.

For me, in those early college trips, psychedelics were more intellectual fun and games with my friends rather than internal, spiritual experiences. When the '60s faded into the '70s and I left college to pursue my graduate studies, I left that circle of friends and drifted away from my use of psychedelics. This wasn't due to any bad experiences or an active turning away, but rather a lack of opportunity coupled with lack of driving desire. Even so, I remained interested in the phenomenon. Although I wasn't in that world anymore, I knew that world continued to exist, through the occasional news reports of "two million hits of LSD seized." I knew that somebody—many somebodies—must still be taking psychedelics.

As I finally came to consider my first MDMA trip, unlike my college days, my first step was to go to the New York Public Library and look up the research on MDMA. In 1990, there was very little published in the medical literature on the use of MDMA in humans. However, the little information I did find convinced me that MDMA was safe when it actually was MDMA, when it was taken in a single dose, and when the user was adequately hydrated.

Profile: Alexander T. "Sasha" Shulgin, Ph.D., and Ann Shulgin

Sasha and Ann Shulgin are extraordinary individuals. Sasha, a chemist with an early interest in mescaline and other hallucinogens, began his career at Dow Chemical in the early 1960s where he developed a financially successful product and was rewarded with support to explore whatever he wanted. Even so, shortly thereafter he left Dow Chemical, all licenses in hand, to create the world's quirkiest backyard Schedule I drug laboratory. In this lab, Shulgin has created and tested hundreds of novel psychedelics, sharing his discoveries with the U.S. government and with the public. How does one test a new, still-legal psychedelic, when the lab animals given it simply stare at the wall for eight hours? With self-experimentation, that's how—by the creator and a few intrepid friends: poets, chemists, therapists, and others, with the single requirement of a report on their experience.

Ann is an extraordinary psychotherapist who provides deep, heartfelt guidance and assistance to troubled travelers and who contributed groundbreaking conceptualizations of the "other" or "shadow" that dwells within us all. Sasha and Ann published their findings (with chemical recipes) in *PIHKAL: Phenethylamines I Have Known and Loved—A Chemical Love Story* and *TIHKAL: Tryptamines I Have Known and Loved—The Continuation* to document Sasha's discoveries and to guarantee that they will never be suppressed. Three years aftern *PIHKAL* was published, the Feds changed their mind about Sasha. The Drug Enforcement Administration (DEA) raided Sasha's lab and demanded he turn over his DEA license. Sasha and Ann are incisive and loving voices within the psychedelic community, as well as harsh critics of the federal government's irrational drug policy on information dissemination, research process, and clinical practice.

As busy as they are, Sasha and Ann always took the time to respond to e-mails from "that psychologist from New York City interested in psychedelics." Sasha and Ann have sat on numerous panels I've convened at conferences, and they never fail to draw the largest crowds. Sasha (in his early eighties) and Ann (in her late seventies) are the revered patriarch and matriarch of the psychedelic community.

My first experience with MDMA was very positive. I felt increased empathy for myself and for those I love. Usually, when we attempt to go inside—to be introspective—we go only so far before fear of painful knowledge triggers our defenses. With MDMA, empathy increases dramatically, relaxing our defenses and enabling us to continue our introspection much more deeply, bringing us closer to the ground of our being—to our soul. When MDMA is used by a couple, this increase in empathy enables them to get past the hurts and resentments that so often build up in long-term relationships (or that we can bring with us, as childhood baggage, even into new relationships). We are reminded of why we came to love our mate in the first place, seeing ourselves, our partners, and the relationship unvarnished yet with deep compassion and acceptance.

I had that type of experience, and it enabled me to feel safe in considering use of the classic hallucinogens such as LSD and psilocybin-containing mushrooms. Specifically, this positive experience with MDMA helped me feel comfortable taking LSD for the first time in nineteen years (as described above in "The Mother of All Trips").

Profile: Timothy Leary, Ph.D.; Oscar "Oz" Janiger, Ph.D.; Betty Eisner, Ph.D.

In October 1995, the Drug Policy Foundation (now called the Drug Policy Alliance) held its annual conference in Santa Monica, California. I chaired a panel called "Regulating Psychedelic Drugs," featuring "A Brief History of Psychedelics Research," by me; "Pre-regulation, Restriction, and Prohibition," by Alexander "Sasha" Shulgin; "Recent Developments in Psychiatric Research," by Charles Grob; and "Scenarios for the Future," by Rick Doblin. It was also the weekend of Timothy Leary's last birthday party.

During the afternoon after my panel, Rick Doblin asked me if I was available to accompany Betty Eisner, Ph.D., one of the early psychedelic researchers from the L.A. area, who needed some assistance getting around. Having just read about her pioneering research (with Sidney Cohen and with Oz Janiger), I was thrilled to spend some quality time with Eisner. We spent the afternoon together at the conference and later at her home. Afterward, Eisner asked me if I wanted to come to a dinner party at Oz Janiger's home, after which we would all go to Tim Leary's seventy-fifth birthday party. I was in heaven!

The parties at Janiger's and at Leary's homes were wonderful, in large part because I got to talk with many of the researchers I'd only been reading about until that point. In addition to Eisner and Janiger, I met Ram Dass (the former Richard Alpert, Ph.D., who was Leary's colleague at Harvard) and many others, but the height of the evening for me came when I had some time alone with Leary.

By chance, I came across Leary, in his then-trademark zebra-print sport coat and with a beautiful young girl on each arm (in reality, helping to steady him in the advanced stages of the prostate cancer that would kill him six months later), talking with another man I didn't know. I joined them and watched as a nitrous oxide balloon was passed. I noted that Leary put it to his lips, but did not inhale. Eventually, the man left and the girls wandered off, and for a few minutes, Leary and I were alone.

I pulled out a joint, lit it, and offered it to him, and this time, he did inhale. As we smoked, I told him how much I liked his beautiful work with psilocybin before he encountered LSD. I then told him how I especially appreciated his early, prepsychedelic research on reducing the dichotomy between researcher and subject, or doctor and patient, which I knew was why, ten years later at Harvard, he'd taken psychedelics with his experimental subjects—not to "get high," but to have more empathy for what the subjects reported.

Holding the joint in one hand and placing his other hand on my shoulder, in one of the most chillingly obligating statements I've ever been given, Leary locked his eyebrows, looked me directly in the eyes, and said, "It's up to you now."

As I continued to explore my soul and my personality through the powerful tool of psychedelics, I came to prefer *Psilocybe* mushrooms to LSD. I found mushrooms to be gentler and less directive than LSD. I found it reassuring that one of the first signs of psilocybin taking effect is yawning. At that point, 1994 or so, at the age of forty-three, I tripped about once a month, usually taking around 3 dried grams of *Psilocybe cubensis,* always alone and always horizontal—under a blanket on the couch or curled up in bed—with a pad and pen by my side and no music, which I found distracting. I would go inside, always finding and touching the ground of my being before trying to do any psychological analysis. Each trip provided a revealing, realigning contact with the part of me underlying—prior to—my psychology, from which vantage point I would then see my personality with compassion, empathy, acceptance, and love. In each experience I cried—tears for the way I'd lived my life, the ways I'd wasted opportunities for love and growth, the beauty at my core—and I took away the knowledge that the only thing "wrong" with me was that I felt there was something wrong with me. After each experience, I was reinvigorated to pursue the goals and direction I'd crafted for my life.

Profile: Rick Doblin, Ph.D.

Rick Doblin began his career in psychedelics in 1984 by helping to organize the psychedelic community's legal response to the DEA's efforts to criminalize MDMA. The DEA had declared MDMA a Schedule I drug, despite a DEA Administrative Law Judge (ALJ) recommendation that MDMA's legal, therapeutic use be sustained. In 1986, in order to sponsor research under a Food and Drug Administration (FDA) IND (Investigational New Drug) application, Doblin founded the Multidisciplinary Association for Psychedelic Studies (MAPS; www .maps.org), of which he is the executive director.

Summarizing Doblin's extraordinary accomplishments would be impossible in the available space. He is the person most responsible for opening up the government's attitude toward new psychedelic research. MAPS is the only membership-based, nonprofit psychedelic and medical marijuana research organization. MAPS also works on policy issues related to the scientific research with Schedule I drugs.

Doblin's goal is to bring MDMA to market as a prescription medicine administered under the supervision of trained and licensed therapists. He is an energetic advocate for and sponsor of many of the current fledgling psychedelic research projects. MAPS is also focused on harm-reduction efforts within psychedelic culture, at large festivals, and music gatherings, with MAPS Deputy Director Valerie Mojeiko organizing and training teams of "sanctuary" volunteers to offer support to people having difficult psychedelic experiences. MAPS is also pioneering therapist training/research protocols that permit trainees to volunteer to receive one MDMA session in a therapeutic/research setting—receiving the same drug they will be administering to others. Internationally, through multiple visits to the Middle East, Rick is also working to foster cross-national scientific collaboration in Israel and Jordan through the use of MDMA-assisted psychotherapy for post-traumatic stress disorder. Can the day be far away when enemy combatants receive MDMA and begin the process of developing empathy for each other?

One of my goals had become the desire—a sense of urgency—to share my knowledge about psychedelic therapy with others. I felt as if psychedelics were a boon (in the spiritual terms I was beginning to become comfortable with, a "blessing") to me and I felt a beautiful obligation to help by sharing this good news with others. As I began to re-craft my life, I reached out to professors and others in psychedelic-friendly professional settings to see what was out there that might enable me to use my background and knowledge to launch a new career—a new professional Neal more in harmony with the new me emerging in my heart and mind. I wondered where to go for additional training, whether I could find a new job in this fascinating field, whether there might be research utilization consulting opportunities with the new research studies that were beginning to emerge.

As I began to read voraciously in the field of psychedelic research, one of the first books I encountered was *Psychedelic Drugs Reconsidered,* by Lester Grinspoon, M.D., and James Bakalar, of Harvard Medical School and Harvard Law School, respectively, which is still the best, most-accessible introduction to psychedelics history, research, medicine, and societal implications (including a chapter on dangers and a sixty-page annotated bibliography).

Through my reading and surfing on the still-new World Wide Web, I came to know a whole new network of psychedelic researchers, such as chemist Alexander "Sasha" Shulgin, who had created hundreds of novel psychedelics; Rick Doblin, an activist who had founded the Multidisciplinary Association for Psychedelic Studies; John Halpern, a research psychiatrist at Harvard Medical School who was publishing careful, groundbreaking papers in the area; Rick Strassman, another psychiatrist, who had spent six years winding his way through the regulatory thicket to become the first person in a generation to obtain permission to conduct research using psychedelics with human subjects, and many, many others. The early '90s saw the dawn of the Internet, and each of these individuals was amazingly responsive to my inquiries and requests for information to feed my still-early knowledge of the field. Several are now much-loved friends.

Over the years since then, I've learned a lot about helping the field forward, and I have been extremely gratified to help the research become more accepted through a combination of public speaking, including Grand Rounds at Memorial Sloan-Kettering Cancer Center on the use of hallucinogens with the dying, at New York Hospital on the state of the art in psychedelic research, at NYU on rescheduling psychedelics, and at many Evening Talks at the New York Open Center (special thanks to J. P. Harpignes and Ralph White for inviting me); conference work, including curation and master of ceremonies (e.g., at the annual *Horizons: Perspectives on Psychedelics* conference and at the 2010 MAPS-sponsored *Psychedelic Science in the Twenty-First Century* conference); and publishing (see www.nealgoldsmith.com/psychedelics for a complete list of my publications and presentations).

Profile: Myron Stolaroff, Ph.D.

Myron Stolaroff was an engineer by training, and perhaps it was his practical, geeky mind that enabled him to experience the power of LSD to transform personality. After receiving LSD in 1956 from Al Hubbard (the "Johnny Appleseed" of LSD in the 1950s), Stolaroff established the International Foundation for Advanced Study in Menlo Park, California. The Foundation eventually conducted some 350 LSD and mescaline sessions, including landmark research into the effect of psychedelics on creativity. Stolaroff was a thoughtful commentator and, later, an elder statesman, urging a thoughtful and meditative mind-set, rather than a recreational approach to these sacraments. His books include *The Secret Chief*, an influential biography of psychologist Leo Zeff, Ph.D., who, despite the difficulties arising from the criminalization of psychedelic drugs in the mid-1960s and 1970s, and of MDMA in 1985, continued to work with psychedelics, training a generation of therapists in their use.

In fact, it was following one of my early speaking engagements ("Psychedelic Psychotherapy and Spirituality: New Research, Ancient Practice," presented to the Association for Spirituality and Psychotherapy) that I finally settled in to my current professional focus. I had had a glorious time, presenting to therapists and healers who, while alternative in their therapeutic orientation, for the most part had little or no knowledge of the history of clinical research on psychedelics or their therapeutic applications.* I had received a standing ovation and

*One senior member even came dressed up in "hippie" garb: bell-bottom pants, granny glasses, flowered shirt, beads, and the like. When I expressed my dismay—that he was trivializing this profound area of research and practice—he flashed me the peace sign and responded, "Mellow out, man. You're bringing me down! Isn't that what you're going to be talking about?" By the end of my presentation, however, he understood the profound nature of this research.

was riding home in a taxi, telling my wife about this wonderful evening. She said to me, "Let me get this straight: you presented what you are passionate about to other psychologists and you were lovingly received. So what is it that's keeping you from finally and completely leaving the world of business and re-launching your psychotherapy practice?" I was overwhelmed with love and gratitude for my wife—and with relief—and I determined to do exactly that. I resolved to get additional training (I chose yoga psychotherapy, Psychosynthesis, and Imago Relationship Therapy) and ultimately reopened the clinical practice I'd closed after my stint working with Ted Smith during and after getting my master's degree from NYU, when I left for California to pursue my applied research doctorate at Claremont Graduate University.

Profile: John H. Halpern, M.D.

As I continued to explore the research literature, I saw a very interesting article on the use of hallucinogens in the treatment of addiction by a new researcher in the field, John H. Halpern, M.D., at that point (the early 1990s) still a psychiatry resident at Harvard Medical School.[3] As I read, I found point after point that matched my own thinking, and, in my enthusiasm, I picked up the phone and called Halpern at Harvard. He answered the phone, we had a wonderful conversation, and, over the years, John has become a dear friend and colleague (and contributor of the foreword to this book).

Halpern has conducted and published much important psychedelic research at Harvard. His research portfolio includes the use of MDMA for end-stage cancer patients, the neurocognitive and psychological competence of members of the Native American Church (who are legally entitled to use the psychedelic cactus peyote in their religious ceremonies) compared with alcoholic Navajo nonmembers and non-drug-using control Navajo nonmembers, and a similar, very important National Institute on Drug Abuse–funded project just completed on pure Ecstasy users ("pure" Ecstasy users don't use any other drug and are rare, in that most users of illegal drugs also use other illegal drugs, such as marijuana, which contaminates findings on the effect of Ecstasy alone. Halpern found them in Utah teens who used Ecstasy when they danced at raves). Halpern filed an *amicus curiae* brief to the U.S. Supreme Court in the União do Vegetal (Centro Espírita Beneficente União do Vegetal or UDV) ayahuasca religious freedom case, and he has worked from the beginning on the Santo Daime religious freedom case, for which he wrote cogent, at times scathing, rebuttals to the positions of the Department of Justice and the DEA. The Santo Daime case went to trial in 2008 in Oregon with Dr. Halpern as the star witness and achieved complete victory over the U.S. government's attempt to suppress this legitimate church's right to freedom of religion. (Halpern has also been a controversial figure for some in the psychedelic community, due to unproved accusations that he is an ongoing informant against the community, starting with Leonard Pickard, who was convicted of manufacturing LSD.)

As you might imagine, my new practice was radically different from the one I had as a master's level psychological counselor during my NYU years. Rather than the Rogerian therapist I was trained as—I refer to that now as "that annoying kind of therapist"—who mirrors back what the client has said and says, "Go on," I became a very active, personally involved psychotherapist, when appropriate sharing information about my own relationships and life struggles as examples for my clients.

Profile: Ethan Nadelmann, Ph.D.

In 1988, Ethan Nadelmann, a brilliant, fiery Princeton political science professor, had the good fortune to be published on the right topic, in the right journal, at the right moment—that being the same spring issue of the journal *Foreign Policy* as billionaire libertarian financier George Soros. Soros liked Nadelmann's article so much that he eventually persuaded him to leave Princeton to found a Soros-funded drug policy organization, named by Nadelmann, The Lindesmith Center (after Alfred Lindesmith, the first prominent professor to challenge America's drug policies). Among other important projects, The Lindesmith Center convened a monthly drug policy seminar featuring presentations by many leading drug policy professionals, including, from the field of psychedelic research and therapy, Ram Dass, Tom Roberts, Jay Stevens, and Myron Stolaroff in the field of psychedelic research and therapy.

Nadelmann is America's leading voice for drug policy reform. The mission of his current organization, the Drug Policy Alliance, is "to advance those policies and attitudes that best reduce the harms of both drug misuse and drug prohibition, and to promote the sovereignty of individuals over their minds and bodies."*

*From the Drug Policy Alliance Web site: www.drugpolicy.org/about/mission.

I'm convinced that the most important reason for this difference in approach was that I was now using psychedelics for self-inquiry and coming to see myself and my personality very differently and, in some ways, to see myself for the first time. My psychedelically facilitated introspection had brought me to see personality development in a fundamentally new and more detailed way. My experience of the "ground of my being" had convinced me that we are all, in essence, perfect at birth and that underneath our external, acquired, strategic personalities, we are all still fundamentally perfect. I use the word *fundamentally* here to distinguish from the sense of perfection as regular, unblemished, right-angled, and always correct. Rather, I came to see our core perfection in the same sense that every tree in a forest is fundamentally perfect. Each individual tree may have broken branches, wind-driven skewing, lightning strikes, and even mold or other disease, but when you look at the forest as a whole, it becomes clear that these deviations in form are natural and that each individual is a necessary part of a balanced whole and so, in that sense, every tree is perfect, and, in that sense, every human—warts and all—is perfect as well. We are all leaves on the tree of life, sending our energy back toward the center of the tree. Our children are also like leaves on the tree of life, supporting that core of love and life. The leaves will drop off eventually, but the flow of life in the universe will continue. The best way to support the tree of life is to love everyone and everything.

Profile: Rick Strassman, M.D.

Rick Strassman is a psychiatrist who has worked to study psychedelics since he was a college student watching his roommates grapple with these fascinating substances. After medical school and residency, he undertook a six-and-a-half-year odyssey through the federal bureaucracy to become the first person in a generation to obtain permission to conduct psychedelic research with human subjects. Was Strassman given permission to conduct groundbreaking clinical research on psychedelic therapy? Of course not! The government permitted only basic dose-response studies—what's the least amount detectable? What's the most that's tolerable?—which had been done in the 1950s, but were not up to today's technological, methodological, and ethical standards. So Strassman gathered research subjects who were already sophisticated with the study drug, N,N-Dimethyltryptamine, or DMT (selected because it is completely resolved in less than thirty minutes and has been a less notorious psychedelic than LSD), and gave them small and then very large doses, giving white knuckles (as the subjects held on to their grasp on reality) to even the most experienced among the subjects.

All was proceeding well in Strassman's career plan until the national hierarchy of his Buddhist order found out about his research (Strassman was a practicing Buddhist). Fearful for a host of reasons, the order specifically was concerned that the ego death experience from psychedelics might end up confusing the user later during the critical forty-nine-day bardo period immediately following their actual physical death. The order gave Strassman an ultimatum: either stop your research or quit the temple. Strassman quit his research for several years, to write and clarify his thinking.

One of Strassman's most challenging findings has to do with alien abduction. A large proportion of Strassman's subjects interpreted their DMT experiences as including interaction with an alien entity, most often experienced as a creature from another part of the universe, an alternate universe, or another dimension. Strassman doesn't second-guess his subjects and dutifully reports these experiences as described; he has written a second book speculating that the psychedelic dimension would be a much more efficient way to "travel" around the universe than spacecraft. Strassman is now conducting psychedelic research again, primarily looking at ayahuasca this time.

It was this psychedelically derived vision of the perfect "ground of our being"—the psyche—that helped me to see that neurosis is a misnomer (literally a "wrong name") and that all of us garden-variety neurotics are fundamentally healthy, like a forest is healthy, if struggling, and that psychology had betrayed its roots in the study of the psyche, or soul, and in its quest for medical legitimacy, had pathologized normal development. Each of us faces the brick walls of our developmental challenges, and the task for each of us is to recognize that these developmental barriers are not infinitely high, but we can get up over them, climb up to the next level. Then the developmental barriers are most accurately and therefore most effectively seen as the vertical portion of a step. Development can't proceed at a consistent 45-degree slope, but rather moves more stepwise: easy horizontal progress becoming a vertical wall (a period of extremely rapid growth). Step after step we go through relatively flat, easy, stable periods that rather abruptly become transformative times—vertical walls that require persistence and bravery to overcome. As Jean Piaget demonstrated for cognitive development, psychological maturity develops through distinct stages, in a stepwise fashion. Overcoming the neurotic obstacles of childhood results in maturation and, through various stages, ultimately to wisdom.[4] Since no one has EVER had perfect parents, everyone must face and overcome (or avoid) those developmental walls in a beautiful, natural, developmental process.

It was this perspective on our essential Ok-ness that inspired my clinical philosophy.

Profile: Robert S. Gable, Ed.D., Ph.D., J.D.

Bob Gable was the advisor I was assigned when I arrived at Claremont Graduate School for my doctoral program. The expectation was that students would switch advisors once they found their research area of interest. Gable was interested in the built environment, drug policy, social applications of operant conditioning, and legal issues. I was interested in the diffusion of innovation, research utilization, and bureaucratic change, with a decidedly humanistic bent, but Gable—brilliant, intellectually demanding, and a fiercely independent thinker—provided me with astute guidance as I navigated my way through the doctoral program.

Years after graduation, I was reading a footnote in an annotated bibliography in an out-of-print journal—the epitome of obscure knowledge—when I came across a reference to an article listing the authors as Leary, T., Metzner, R., Presnell, M., Weil, G., Schwitzgebel, R., and Kinne, S. Although by then most people knew Bob as Bob Gable, during the period I was at Claremont, for reasons of ease of use, he had changed his name, switching to Gable from Schwitzgebel. I immediately called him on the telephone and sure enough, he and his twin brother, Kirkland (who simultaneously changed his name to Gable with Bob and is also a psychologist and attorney), had indeed done research with Leary's group at Harvard. It took ten years after I left graduate school for me to more fully understand the connection I had with this wonderful, reluctant mentor.

As my practice grew, so did I. I became involved in many professional activities that formed naturally in this exciting intellectual and spiritual context.

In 2001, with a partner, Ed Rosenfeld, I created the Poetry Science Talks (PST) salon discussion group—an ongoing series of out-of-box discussions and good fellowship. Poetry Science Talks is actually not about poetry or science, but rather focuses on a poetical science (and philosophy) broad enough to accommodate—and integrate—seeming opposites: of science and art, mind and body, matter and energy, spirit and flesh. We meet monthly and have had more than one hundred soulful, integral talks on creative media, ecology and governance, healing, philosophy of mind, post-postmodern science and technologies, and everything in between.

Profile: Thomas Roberts, Ph.D.

Tom Roberts is a communications hub of the psychedelic research community. A retired psychology professor and cofounder (with Bob Jesse) of the Center for Spiritual Practices (www.csp.org), Roberts created and teaches the first U.S. college-level catalogue-listed course on psychedelics. He is the author of several books on the subject and most recently was coeditor (with Michael Winkelman) of *Psychedelic Medicine: New Evidence for Hallucinogenic Substances as Treatments,* the first textbook on psychedelics in forty years. Roberts' influential e-mail distribution is read by every in-touch professional in the psychedelic community.

My interest with PST was in a broader understanding of reality than can be attained through either the poetical perspective on reality, such as creativity, intuition, and spirituality, or the scientific perspective, the realms of the physical, matter, and logic. The "Poetry Science" perspective represents a third, transcendent view of reality that might be labeled integral science and philosophy—a worldview that can serve as a conceptual umbrella for quantum mechanics, meditation, emergent properties, psychedelics, cosmology, placebo, relativity, spontaneous remission, governance, stigmata, artificial intelligence, healing, peak experience, psychosomatics, innovation, and that spark of knowing insight.

Profile: Roland R. Griffiths, Ph.D.

Roland Griffiths is a professor of behavioral biology and of neuroscience at the Johns Hopkins University School of Medicine. Griffiths is nearing the peak of his career, having published dozens of peer-reviewed, drug policy research studies in prestigious behavioral pharmacology medical journals, on substances such as caffeine and benzodiazepines. Many of his studies have been funded by the Drug Enforcement Administration. In 2006, Griffiths came out with a paper titled "Psilocybin Can Occasion Mystical Experiences Having Substantial and Sustained Personal Meaning and Spiritual Significance." For a professional with less stature, that could have been a career killer, but for Griffiths, it occasioned the most positive accompanying commentary possible, and from drug warriors at that (e.g., a former director of the National Institute on Drug Abuse), praising the methodological rigor of his study. It seems that Griffiths, a long-time meditator, was contacted by Bob Jesse of the Council on Spiritual Practices, and had become interested in the spiritual effects of psychedelics—and had the seniority to research it. The study was important for many reasons, not the least being that it was conducted on a normal, nonclinical population; its release in 2006 was a turning point in credibility for the entire field of psychedelic research.

In addition, I began to volunteer at the "chill tent" at Burning Man, called Sanctuary. Most people think of Burning Man (the annual art installation "happening" in the Nevada desert that draws some fifty thousand visitors for the week leading up to Labor Day) as a psychedelic bacchanalia, an autonomous free zone where everyone is in costumes, creating fire, tripping, and having sex all day and all night. In fact, for many this is the case, but when one looks a bit deeper, beyond the loud flash of garish makeup, ubiquitous flames and explosions, and the incessant, deafening techno beat, one finds an extraordinary undergirding of people in service, a dharmic network of selflessness that is sometimes difficult to see but always present.

Profile: Stephen Ross, M.D.; Anthony P. Bossis, Ph.D.; Jeffrey R. Guss, M.D.

In February 2006, I gave a talk at the New York Open Center called "The Ten Lessons of Psychedelic Therapy, Rediscovered." The next morning, I received a very enthusiastic e-mail from Steve Ross, a young, accomplished NYU psychiatrist, telling me about his plans for a psychedelic research project at the NYU School of Medicine and asking if I would speak to his new psychedelic discussion group at the hospital. I was honored and of course agreed. Actually, I felt intimidated at the prospect of speaking to a formal group of psychiatry professors. When I arrived however, PowerPoint presentation in hand, I found that I already knew all the members of Ross's group, each of whom had attended talks I'd given or had otherwise become colleagues.

After a great conversation with Ross, we parted as new friends, and I've been pleased to informally consult on the project ever since. In April 2008, I was honored to be invited to give the first NYU Medical Center, Division of Alcoholism and Drug Abuse, Psychedelic Grand Rounds, titled "Rescheduling Psychedelics: Recent History and Scenarios for the Future." That September, Professors Ross, Bossis, and

Guss gave the 2009 Season Opener presentation at my Poetry Science Talks salon, and less than a month later, Dr. Ross presented on the NYU Psilocybin Cancer Research and Education Project at the 2009 Horizons: Perspectives on Psychedelics conference in New York.

All of this came after an early period of uncertainty, during which the viability of the project was repeatedly threatened. Thankfully, the NYU Psilocybin Cancer Research and Education Project is now well established and has become an important example of the mainstreaming of psychedelic research. With clinical research projects using psychedelics under way or completed at the medical schools of Johns Hopkins, Harvard, UCLA, and NYU, among others, the focus of psychedelic policy activism has shifted from gaining permission to conduct preclinical studies, and Phase 0 (single subtherapeutic doses of the study drug to 10–15 subjects) and Phase I (20–80 subject) trials. The emphasis is now on gathering the data to justify Phase II (100–300 subject) clinical trials and the large-scale, multisite Phase III studies needed to prove safety and efficacy for each clinical indication tested, as required for FDA approval to market new drugs.

Sanctuary is a safe haven for people who are having a difficult time—either a psychedelic emergency or, as I prefer to characterize it, a spiritual emergence, or perhaps just too much Burning Man (the heat, the dust, the crowds, the tentmates . . .). It is a place where people can behave in ways—speaking or crying incoherently; being unresponsive—that could get them sedated by the medical team or even ejected from Burning Man, were they to do so on the Playa.* Not all, or even most, Sanctuary volunteers are therapists back in the

---

*Playa: "A dry lake bed at the bottom of a desert basin, sometimes temporarily covered with water. Playas have no vegetation and are among the flattest geographical features in the world." (*The American Heritage Science Dictionary* [2005, Houghton Mifflin Company] ed., s.v. "Playa.") *Playa* is the word Burners use to refer to the yellow-dust desert on which the Burning Man community is built each year.

"default world" (Burners' way of referring to the "real" world of work and family—the other fifty-one weeks of the year), but all are soulfully therapeutic. There is a screening and then a training process, and as a result, Sanctuary volunteers tend to be a loving, giving, empathic group, and it is a pleasure to work with them. It's also hugely rewarding—an honor—to work with those Burners who drop in for support or a safe space to unfold his process. Working at Sanctuary isn't about conducting psychotherapy—there is no time for ongoing therapeutic intervention—but is everything about creating a safe container or nest for the drop-in to complete their process, whatever (short of violence) it may be.

In one instance, a reveler was dancing around the Playa, naked and crying and bumping into others, but unable to speak. This person's friends were concerned that he might be ejected, as he was somewhat disruptive, but he was noncommunicative, and so they brought him to Sanctuary. We found this person to be nonviolent and simply accepted his unusual behavior, providing soothing support until he began to come down and was able to speak again, at which point he departed Sanctuary on his own (he would not wait for his friends to come pick him up). As the theme of Burning Man is radical self-reliance, it is not the job of the Sanctuary worker to ensure the safety of departing Sanctuary visitors, but just to enable them to "do their thing"—that includes departing—in a safe, supportive environment.

Another instance was a young woman who came in describing herself as having taken "a little too much mushrooms." As I spoke quietly with her, she would occasionally blurt out a string of guttural expletives. After the second occurrence I asked her about it, and she explained that she had Tourette's Syndrome and was off her medication. When I asked her why she wasn't taking her medication, she explained that she had tried dozens of different medications, from neuroleptics to stimulants, but that each had debilitating side effects that she felt were worse than the Tourette's symptoms. She told me that, in fact, her symptoms only emerged when she was anxious, but that she lived with calm, loving roommates and so she generally didn't need medication at home. She had decided to continue her nondrug approach at Burning Man, even though the atmosphere was tense for her, and so her symptoms had reemerged. She was simply enjoying her mushroom trip while ignoring or tolerating her Tourette's symptoms. For the rest of her several-hours stay at Sanctuary, we spoke about her mind and spirit, punctuated from time to time by an outburst of tics and expletives, which we both happily ignored. An uplifting and empowering experience for us both, I believe.

Profile: Bob Jesse

One of the first places I encountered as I surfed the nascent Internet was the Council on Spiritual Practices (CSP), founded by Bob Jesse, a former Oracle executive, who has been extremely influential in shifting the positioning of psychedelics from treating pathology to a sacramental approach not necessarily requiring medical supervision. I was intrigued by his idea to analyze all prior Supreme Court rulings on religious freedom defenses in drug cases, to "reverse engineer" a set of spiritual practices that could withstand court scrutiny. Through CSP, Jesse and his colleagues recently initiated a study, conducted at Johns Hopkins and reported around the world, of the psychospiritual effects of psilocybin in healthy volunteers (csp.org/psilocybin). This expands the emphasis in hallucinogen research beyond the medical treatment of ill people to include the betterment of well people, contributing to a science of pro-social development.

In 1995, at the CSP conference "Psychoactive Sacraments," Jesse met Johns Hopkins psychologist Bill Richards, who had worked as a psychedelic guide during the prior wave of research at Spring Grove and Maryland Psychiatric Institute in the late 1960s and early 1970s. In January 1996, at a CSP steering committee meeting in the Maslow room at Esalen, a multidisciplinary group of fifteen leaders (including Huston Smith, Brother David Steindl-Rast, Willis Harman, and Bob Schuster) identified it as a goal to assess with modern methods and measures and to publish new data on the safety and spiritual import of psilocybin in healthy, normal volunteers. Some months after that meeting, former NIDA director Bob Schuster introduced Jesse to Rowland Griffiths, Ph.D. (an influential professor of behavior biology and of neuroscience at the Johns Hopkins University School of Medicine Shuster felt very sure that they should meet). Griffiths and Jesse corresponded, spoke by phone, and before long met in Baltimore. CSP convened three-day science meetings in February 1998 and March 2000 to explore scientific and regulatory feasibility and to begin to develop a research approach and Griffiths and Jesse began sketching the design of a study of psilocybin in healthy normals. It was important from CSP's perspective to highlight scientist and guide as separate roles and skills. At that point, Jesse introduced Griffiths and Richards. As a Hopkins study grew more likely, funding commitments began to come in through CSP.

I find it delightful that while his formal training is in engineering, Bob is also co-convener of a spiritual community formed around ecstatic dance!

Yet another example of the broad, elastic nest provided at Sanctuary occurred when a couple came in under the influence of Bromo-DragonFLY (Bromo-benzodifuranyl-isopropylamine), a very potent and long-lasting (up to several days) phenylethylamine (commonly referred to as a phenethylamine) psychedelic. When friends brought them in at the beginning of my 6 p.m. to 12 a.m. shift, neither one could speak effectively, and they were laid down on separate cots to ride it out. I sat with both of them, on and off, for the next six hours and then left them in other loving hands. The next day, I had the same shift, and upon my arrival they were still there, only he was in a bad state, moaning and crying out. Others were sitting with them at that point, so during that shift, I simply observed from afar. The next day, my shift was from 12 p.m. to 6 p.m., and when I arrived, I learned that they had just departed

Sanctuary—shaky, but happy—no more than an hour before. That meant that they had spent approximately thirty-six hours going through a very difficult and prolonged experience—and coming to resolution— in the kindly, safe space provided by Sanctuary. If they had simply been on the Playa or in their tent with their friends, they could very likely have been taken away in an ambulance—an expensive, unnecessary end (especially as sedatives would have been administered) that wouldn't have enabled them to fully experience and, importantly, to resolve their journey. That is why we call this very special place Sanctuary.

Another extracurricular activity I've been drawn to in recent years is curating and hosting the annual Horizons: Perspectives on Psychedelics conference (www.horizonsnyc.org), held on the NYU campus in New York City in late September annually since 2007. Horizons is a research-focused conference. (After all, how much can attendees get from yet another war story about how "tripped out" someone got or how much they experienced God at the concert last weekend?) Over the past few years, conference organizer Kevin Balktick and I have been able to host an extraordinary roster of the leaders in the field of psychedelic research, including those shown in the box below.

Horizons: Perspectives on Psychedelics Conference Speakers, 2007–2010

- *Kenneth Alper, M.D.*, associate professor, NYU Medical Center (Psychiatry and Neurology); ibogaine expert
- *Allan Hunt Badiner*, author, editor, *Zig Zag Zen*
- *John Perry Barlow*, author, lyricist, essayist, and cofounder of the Electronic Frontier Foundation
- *Mary P. Cosimano, MSW*, graduate social worker, Department of Psychiatry and Behavioral Sciences, Johns Hopkins University School of Medicine
- *Alicia Danforth*, clinical psychedelic researcher, UCLA cancer anxiety trial

▶ *Erik Davis*, author, Nomad Codes: Adventures in Modern Esoterica, TechGnosis, and The Visionary State

▶ *Rick Doblin, Ph.D.*, founder and executive director, Multidisciplinary Association for Psychedelic Studies (MAPS)

▶ *Earth and Fire Erowid*, cofounders, www.erowid.org

▶ *Robert Forte*, author, editor, *Entheogens and the Future of Religion*

▶ *Neal M. Goldsmith, Ph.D.*, author and psychotherapist

▶ *Alex and Allyson Grey*, visionary artists

▶ *Roland R. Griffiths, Ph.D.*, professor in the departments of psychiatry and neurosciences at the Johns Hopkins University School of Medicine

▶ *Charles S. Grob, M.D.*, professor of psychiatry and pediatrics at the UCLA School of Medicine and director of the Division of Child and Adolescent Psychiatry at Harbor-UCLA Medical Center

▶ *Jeffrey Guss, M.D.*, clinical assistant professor of psychiatry, New York University School of Medicine, and investigator and director of training, NYU Cancer Anxiety Psilocybin Project

▶ *J. P. Harpignies*, author, editor, conference producer

▶ *Jill Harris*, managing director, Public Policy, Drug Policy Alliance

▶ *Julie Holland, M.D.*, assistant professor of psychiatry, NYU School of Medicine; private practice, New York City

▶ *Bob Jesse*, organizer, Council on Spiritual Practices (csp.org/about)

▶ *Matthew W. Johnson, Ph.D.*, assistant professor, department of Psychiatry and Behavioral Sciences, Johns Hopkins University School of Medicine

▶ *Don Lattin*, author, Harvard Psychedelic Club and freelance journalist

▶ *Andy Letcher, Ph.D.*, author, *Shroom: A Cultural History of the Magic Mushroom*; academic lecturer; folk musician

- *Dan Merkur, Ph.D.,* psychoanalyst in private practice and a research reader in the study of religion at the University of Toronto; author, *The Ecstatic Imagination: Psychedelic Experiences and the Psychoanalysis of Self-Actualization*
- *Michael Mithoefer, M.D.,* former emergency room physician-turned-psychiatrist in private practice, testing MDMA as a treatment for post-traumatic stress disorder
- *Valerie Mojeiko,* deputy director, MAPS
- *Dimitri Mobengo Mugianis,* founding member, Freedom Root, The Ibogaine Project; ibogaine treatment provider; Bwiti initiate and Nganga (apprentice healer)
- *Ethan Nadelmann, Ph.D.,* founder and executive director, Drug Policy Alliance
- *David E. Nichols, Ph.D.,* professor of medicinal chemistry and pharmacology in the School of Pharmacy and Pharmaceutical Sciences at Purdue University; cofounder and director of Preclinical Research, Heffter Institute (www.heffter.org)
- *Annie Oak,* founder of the Women's Visionary Congress and the Women's Entheogen Fund
- *Torsten Passie, M.D., Ph.D.,* assistant professor for Consciousness Studies, Hannover Medical School, Germany
- *Dale Pendell,* author, ethnobotanist, poet
- *Daniel Pinchbeck,* cofounder, *Open City* art/literary journal; author, *2012: The Return of Quetzalcoatl* and *Breaking Open the Head*; editorial director, *Reality Sandwich*
- *Bill Richards, Ph.D.,* psychologist, Psychiatry Department, Johns Hopkins University School of Medicine
- *Ed Rosenfeld, co-librettist with Gerd Stern, reading from their opera, PSYCHE AND DELIA*
- *Stephen Ross, M.D.,* principal investigator, Psilocybin Cancer Project, NYU; assistant professor of psychiatry and oral medicine and director of the Division of Alcoholism and Drug Abuse, Bellevue Hospital; clinical director, NYU Langone

Center of Excellence on Addiction; associate director, Addiction Education, NYU Department of Psychiatry

▶ *Isaiah Saxon and Sean Helfritsch*, lead creative team, Encyclopedia Pictura; creators (while on *Psilocybe* mushrooms) of Bjork's infamous "Wanderlust" 3-D video

▶ *Alexander "Sasha" Shulgin, Ph.D.*, pharmacologist, chemist, and drug developer, and *Ann Shulgin*, lay therapist with psychedelic substances such as MDMA and 2C-B in therapeutic settings while these drugs were still legal. Coauthors of *PiHKAL* and *TiHKAL*.

▶ *Rick Strassman, M.D.*, clinical associate professor of psychiatry, University of New Mexico School of Medicine; author, *DMT-The Spirit Molecule*

▶ *Franz Vollenweider, Ph.D.*, director of the Psychopharmacology and Brain Imaging Research Unit, University Hospital of Psychiatry (Burghölzli); professor of psychiatry, School of Medicine, University of Zurich

▶ *Clare S. Wilkins*, director, Pangea Biomedics ibogaine clinic, Tijuana, Mexico

▶ *Bob Wold*, founder and president of Clusterbusters, Inc., a nonprofit organization that supports research on the use of psilocybin and LSD to treat cluster headaches

The Horizons: Perspectives on Psychedelics conference is a two-day oasis of psychedelic research in the psychedelic desert of contemporary America. Horizons is one of the few opportunities for the psychedelic research community to come together as a community, as well as a rare channel for disseminating state-of-the-art knowledge to the educated-but-amateur civilian interested in this topic. The opportunity to bring in leading psychedelic researchers (and yes, some artists too) to present data, compare notes, and bond socially is both a deep pleasure and a serious responsibility.

Over this entire period, from about 1990 to the present, I've become a frequent speaker on spiritual emergence, resistance to change, drug policy reform, and the integral future of society. Among my publications I am perhaps proudest of "The Ten Lessons of Psychedelic Therapy, Rediscovered" in the recent Praeger textbook, *Psychedelic Medicine*[5]; my affidavit to the California Superior Court in Santa Cruz, "Rescheduling Psilocybin: A Review of the Clinical Research"[6]; and the frequently cited "The Utilization of Policy Research."[7] I've also had the pleasure and the honor (with friend Ed Rosenfeld) of founding and administering several salon discussion groups in New York City.*

I have now become what makes me feel most comfortable in my own skin. As my bio states, I am "a psychotherapist and consultant in private practice, specializing in psychospiritual development—seeing 'neurosis' as the natural unfolding of human maturation. I make use of psychotherapy training in Imago Relationship Therapy; psychosynthesis; yoga psychology; regressive psychotherapies; Rogerian client-centered counseling; and other humanistic, transpersonal, and Eastern traditions (in addition to the lessons found in the research literature on psychedelics). I am also an applied research psychologist and strategic planner working with institutions to foster innovation and change."

Although I think of my transition at that time (around 2001) as reopening the clinical practice I had at the master's level, in fact, my new practice was diametrically different from what I was taught in graduate school. Whereas at the master's level I was taught to passively reflect what the client had said, in my postgraduate training (formal and otherwise) I was being pulled to be myself in session, sharing my own experience and developing a relationship based on trust, through which change could most readily unfold. I had left counseling for corporate

---

*I also helped create quality improvement councils at the American Express Company and AT&T and, while still a graduate student, was an affiliate of the Center for Policy Research at Columbia University, a founder of the Claremont Center for Applied Social Research, and an invited member of the Network of Consultants on Planned Change at the National Institute of Mental Health.

strategic planning, lest I had to found that new school of thought called Kick-in-the-Ass therapy, but now I had found a positive, developmentally oriented practice of acceptance and health.

When I worked at American Express Company during the daytime and at night prepared PowerPoint presentations for talks on the clinical applications of psychedelics, there was a "Day Neal" and a "Night Neal"—my job and my passion were too far apart to fit under the same identity. Now, as a clinician, I can utilize the important lessons provided by psychedelics in the clinical philosophy I develop, and there is just one Neal again.

In looking back, I realize that there has always been this duality between who I felt I was supposed to be and who I knew I really was. The following letter describes a religious experience I had when I was seventeen years old, five months before my first psychedelic experience (at college later that winter). It shows that I had a thoughtful, spiritual orientation before taking psychedelics, and yet this experience faded. Did trying psychedelics six months later enhance that orientation or distract from its unfolding?

A TRUE INTELLECTUAL-RELIGIOUS REVELATION

When Harriet's letter arrived in 2004, I was intrigued to find an old Aerogram folding Air Letter inside, with a note clipped on: "I thought you'd find this interesting—Hq." I quickly saw that it was written by me while in Europe in 1969 when I was seventeen, and sent to her, my high-school sweetheart and still dear friend, back in Great Neck, Long Island.

Dear Harriet,

I am now on the ferry going from Gedser, Denmark, to Travemunde, W. Germany. It vibrates quite a bit. We left our itinerary again, to come south from Oslo, through Copenhagen once again. Next, to Hamburg.

I spoke to you four days ago and have since been too involved in my own thoughts to write you, but now I feel I not only can, but I must.

As you know, I've been doing a lot of thinking lately, and I have been very confused. Even the great peace that I told you of was only a temporary relief. Not only was I thinking about [my older brother and travel-mate's] personality, but also several things in my own head that had been bothering me. This thinking was very scientific (of course), and also very deep and intense, as well as growing rapidly in magnitude. At times, I was convinced I was mad and sometimes (most of the time) I wasn't convinced of anything at all. As I say, all this was growing and growing, until last night, when something truly remarkable happened.

[My brother] and I were with some kids last night, seeing the city; some "underground" night spots—music. Then we left with one of them. We went to a club with good music and the three of us sat down. I started thinking, as I usually do when I hear good music, and I recall now, remarking to myself on the depth and intensity of my thoughts. Then [my brother] got up to go to the bathroom. I started thinking about all the things I had been thinking about this summer. I realized that what I had been doing, basically, was psychoanalyzing myself. The things I saw in my subconscious, the things normally hidden, that I had brought to the surface, sometimes scared me, other times shocked me, but always helped me to realize something about myself. All the incidents and experiences that I've had this summer have all helped me in discovering the secrets of my own head. I got to thinking about how incredible all these things were. It was almost as if it was some master plan I was following. Some real Secret of Life that I was striving so desperately for. And I was, remarkably enough, being shown the way, as if by some Great Force.

Then, all of a sudden, I felt a great energy within me. I thought of the Bible and all the religious precepts that I had learned about yet never really believed. And I understood them, every single one.

I realized how men much wiser and smarter than I could believe in a God. I felt this Energy like an electric shock going through my body. I shook myself several times to see if I was really feeling such a strange thing—and I was! I realized in those few seconds that I was experiencing a true intellectual-religious Revelation. Not just an overwhelming thought, but a true, Bible-like revelation. I felt a presence. An overwhelming feeling that something was showing me the way. I felt as if my life should be devoted to a study of the mind as well as the spirit. I felt a great belief in a Great Force of some kind, a real meaning to life, through the search for meaning. Not a desperate, mazelike search, but an intellectual and spiritual search, in an orderly manner.

I sat back as I felt this force draining out of my body, and with it I felt my strength being drained away also. I was exhausted. I couldn't move a muscle. I felt my chest become lighter and I felt as if a great weight was relieved from it. I was not tired, though, and my mind was exited and alive. I felt as if this were the real thing. In this state of physical exhaustion and mental acuity, I did the logical thing: I rested my body and used my mind. I flashed before me all the things I had been thinking of this summer, all my problems, and they all fell into place. All the problems and puzzles were solved, obvious, and easy to figure out. Actually, all my problems were not solved, as they were the result of a lifetime of experiences, but they were still easy to recognize and see as problems, especially to see what was behind them psychologically.

When [my brother] came back, I tried to tell him about what had just happened. I could still feel a force in my body and so could our friend, because he sat up and tried to find out what was happening. Just before he left, he told me some very interesting things about what he thought of [my brother], (hiding something) and of me (in your brother's shadow), very deep things that I am sure he would not have normally mentioned.

That's the gist of what happened. I am convinced that what I

experienced was real, even monumental. I feel good. I look forward
to studying religion and psychology in school next year. I feel good.
. . . Please don't worry. Everything's cool. See ya soon!

Always yours,

—Neal

After this "true intellectual-religious Revelation" as a seventeen-
year-old in Europe, I got back to the States and the demands of college
(pre-med, I thought). Amazingly, the memory of that overwhelming
experience faded completely away—perhaps *because* it was so overwhelming and outré—and was replaced by my default world (as a Burner
might say). Thirty-five years later, when Harriet gave me back my original Aerogram to her, I immediately remembered the incident and writing about it, and experienced an enormous feeling of waking up to an
earlier self. Through sweat and time, through many detours on my path
and some dead ends, I had finally come back to the "study of the mind,
as well as the spirit," as I felt in that experience that I was meant to. At
precisely that point, thirty-five years later, through the ripening action
of time, American Express, and acid, I was finally, naturally, fulfilling
the vision I'd had so many years ago.

So the intriguing question arises of how change comes about. Does
it unfold gradually, or is it triggered, provoked? Does it ripen? Can it be
sped up? Is fundamental change even possible (or even a useful, healthy
goal)? Those are the topics I will address next.

2

IS FUNDAMENTAL PERSONALITY CHANGE POSSIBLE?

THE CONCEPT OF CHANGE AND ITS ACTION

To provide a firm foundation for our logical analysis of change, let's start by defining the term in its most fundamental sense, in mathematics and physics—but simply—and then work our way up to more complex connotations of change in psychology and human relations.

Perhaps the most basic component of any definition of the term *change* is that change requires the passage of time. Even in a flat line (see figure 2.1), when nothing seems to be changing, the passage of time itself is a change. With a slope (see figure 2.2), we can see change in its continuous, increasing form. In figure 2.3, we see that with great variability, change can still be a net flat slope. With a sine curve (figure 2.4), we've simplified random variation into its simplest net-zero form, but when we increase the slope of the sine curve to 45 degrees (see figure 2.5), the sine curve turns into a stepwise curve. Even more interesting, due to the concavity and convexity around the inflection point of the curve, there is an energy sink on the most horizontal portion of the curve, leading to a certain inertia before great transformative change. Likewise, there is a corresponding overhang—a negative arc at the most vertical portion of the curve—that, like an overhanging ledge

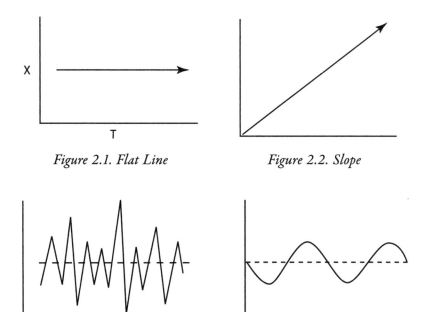

Figure 2.1. Flat Line   Figure 2.2. Slope

Figure 2.3. Static;   Figure 2.4. Sine Curve
No Change in the Real World

mountain climbers sometimes encounter, may seem impossible to get up over, but through a leap of faith or a quantum jump, we can surmount. Of course, when applying these abstract mathematical ideas to our own personal challenges, the way stepwise change works is that once you get over the hump and are on the next higher horizontal section looking back down, the developmental challenge of the prior vertical wall that we were just struggling with so mightily will now seem quite obvious.

Finally, if we make our sine curve completely vertical, widen the top, and narrow the bottom, we have created a spiral (see figure 2.6). The spiral continues the sine curve's undulating variation, but adds another dimension of depth to the model. Interestingly, if the slope of the spiral is great enough, one side's upward swing can be lower than the other side's downward swing. The best example is the Leaning Tower of Pisa, where the lean is so great that as one descends the spiral staircase inside the tower, half the time one is walking upward relative to the earth—ascending on the way down!

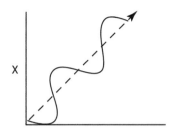

Figure 2.5. Stepwise Development

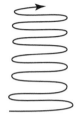

Figure 2.6. Spiral

Many important expressions of nature—our heartbeat, rocking a baby, a musical beat, mantras, counting, breathing—have this same rhythm of sinelike, stepwise transformation rather than unitary, continuous change. We'll return to this essential rhythmicity below.

Change requires the passage of time and often entails rhythmicity, but there's more to change than simple difference or contrast (see figure 2.7). In mythology, the command "Let there be light!" created the first contrast, changing unitary chaos into a duality of light and dark. A checkerboard has difference, but since the elements remain stable—they don't morph from black to white and the squares don't change in shape or size—we don't generally think of a checkerboard as changing. Even so, since at the very least time elapses, it is fair to say that today's checkerboard is a different object from yesterday's checkerboard. Even if it isn't moved, the time and place in space have changed, the checkerboard has aged, faded, and decomposed in subtle ways, and so time alone in some sense equals change.

Growth, then, must entail quantitative change (see figure 2.8); for example, the same black-and-white checkerboard pattern, only with

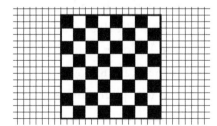

Figure 2.7. Checkerboard

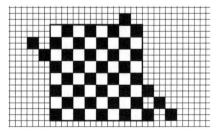

Figure 2.8. Growth

more squares that spread well beyond the traditional 8-inch-by-8-inch checkerboard.

Development (see figure 2.9) entails stepwise change, a progression through a sequence of stages. Development occurs in people, of course, but also in inanimate objects, such as stars, that have a natural, default way of developing in interaction—in sync—with the surrounding ecology.

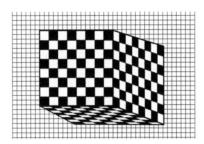

Figure 2.9. Development

How do growth and development differ from maturation? To mature is to change by ripening through a life cycle, and *maturation* is the general term for the natural aging process. Maturation can be seen in the unfolding of stepwise or stagewise development, but there is no maturation implied in the simple quantitative process of growth—becoming more.

It is interesting to note that psychoanalyst Dan Merkur has observed that even spiritual adepts go through a stepwise process of personal development.

THE DEVELOPMENTAL PSYCHOLOGY OF SPIRITUAL EMERGENCE

Dan Merkur considers psychedelics to be a convenient generator of the mystical experience, a helpful aid to both psychoanalysis and spiritual development, but not to be confused with enlightenment itself. In his book, *Ecstatic Imagination,* he writes:

Roberto Assagioli (1991) suggested that spiritual awakening is typically preceded by disaffection with materialism. Concern with the meaning of life may become acute, but may be dismissed as unrealistic. The prospect of change is resisted because it is unknown, feared, and expected to be burdensome in its demands. A spiritual awakening then intervenes. Religious experience, which Assagioli conceived in metaphysical terms, may occur either spontaneously or through earnest desire.

But immediately upon spiritual awakening, the personality may suffer in inflation, self-exaltation, or grandiosity, due to, "confusion between what a person is potentially and what he is actually." Other vicissitudes include emotional excitement and lability, missionary zeal, fanaticism, and an idealism whose futility leads to depression and self-destructive despair. With greater realism the grandiosity subsides and, "a period of joyful inner and external expansion" takes place. "Sometimes it is the mystical aspect and enlightenment which are dominant, in other cases new energies are released in the form of selfless heroic action, benevolent service, or artistic creativity. The former personality with its sharp corners and disagreeable traits has been replaced with a new person, who is full of kindness and sympathy. A person who smiles at us and at the whole world, wanting only to give others pleasure, to be useful, and to share his new spiritual riches, which seem to be overflowing from within."

This period of joyous productivity can last a lifetime, but in most cases it ends in an acute emotional crisis. "The 'old Adam' resurfaces with his habits, tendencies, and passions, and the man now realizes that he has a long, complex, demanding task of purification and transformation ahead of him." The reversion to the prior organization of the personality may cause depression over the loss of joyousness. "Often this general sense of torment is supplemented by a more specific moral crisis: the ethical conscience has been awakened and the person is overcome by a profound sense of guilt or remorse for the wrong they have committed. He then passes a severe judgment on himself." The intensity of the suffering may motivate attempts to deny the value and reality of spiritual transformation. Preoccupation with the internal conflicts may lead to neglect of public concerns, resulting in "unsympathetic and undeserved judgment from his family, friends, and even from his doctors." The adverse criticisms intensify the conflict by encouraging the tendency to denial. "Exhaustion, insomnia, depression, irritability and restlessness, and a variety of physical symptoms" may follow. In other cases premature resolution of the conflict may be attempted through the repression rather than the transformation of the lower aspects of the personality. An exacerbation of the conflict ensues.

The spiritual crisis is resolved through, "assimilation. That is to say the new ideas which have come to enrich the conscious personality to become an integral part of it." However, as the process of spiritual transformation nears completion there sometimes occurs what St. John of the Cross termed the "dark night of the soul." The symptoms include "an emotional sense of deep depression, which may even verge on despair, an acute sense of unworthiness, which in some cases leads to a person feeling himself to be lost or damned. A painful sense of mental impotence. A weakening of the will and of self-control, lack of desire, and a great reluctance to act." The final completion of spiritual transformation is indicated by a "glorious spiritual resurrection that puts an end to every suffering and every disorder . . . and represents the fullness of spiritual health."[1]

There's a big difference between a spiritual experience and a spiritual life. Certainly the experiences that psychedelics provide, while significant, perhaps even uniquely powerful, are generally still transitory unless you have a prepared mind. I think of a life lived as creating compost or humus in which advanced experiences can take root. If a perfect master could touch the forehead of an eight-year-old, youthful and unformed, and instill one minute of enlightenment, over time that experience would fade and so would not have a truly lasting transformative effect on the child's life—even though the person might still remember it. If that same one minute of enlightenment were provided to an older person who's been a meditator for fifty years, it could be the tipping point that initiates profound advancement.

What then do we mean by *transformative change*? In the vernacular, *transformative* implies not just developmental change through stages, but also experiencing novel stages or embarking on a new developmental path (see figure 2.9).

It's clear that change in people is more than the accumulation of more—more data, more facts, more information, even more knowledge. True change that is meaningful to people entails transformation to a new, qualitatively different stage of life, one that is more adaptive, through which more information is processed or information is processed more efficiently. This kind of profound, transformative change may be seen when a caterpillar changes into a chrysalis and then into a butterfly, or when a human embryo is born. Can this kind of transformative change be elicited deliberately?

PERSONALITY DEVELOPMENT AS IMMATURE STRATEGY

What is the current, normal, neurotic situation for most people? We first see a cautious distance, especially in infants, and under that, skepticism and fear. Under that? Pain. And under that? The basic need for love. If we read that sequence in reverse order, we can see the chronology of how it develops: we begin with a natural need for love, but when the family foundation is unsafe, the expectation of love is unfulfilled and pain ensues. When love is not received, skepticism and anxiety become a generalized condition. We form personality in relationship with our parents and, the younger we are the more impressionable we are and the more we are subject to an all-encompassing, immersive, parental ecology.

Imagine a little girl sitting on the floor, making a drawing for Mommy with the full flower of altruism and love in her heart. Beautiful, but in this example, she's drawing with Mommy's lipstick and she's doing it on the dining room wall! Now Mommy walks in the room. What does she do? If Mommy is the Buddha, Mommy notes her emotion with compassion (yes, the Buddha-Mommy still has emotions; she just responds to them with love and acceptance) and gently steers the little girl to a more suitable medium, all the while praising her for her generosity and her artistry. Of course, there are few Buddha-Mommies around, and many of us would respond to a lipstick drawing on the dining room wall with either anger or emotional withdrawal. This is the way certain behaviors in the child—artistic creativity or fearful dependence, for example—are shaped in parent-baby interactions.

In order to understand how the process of personality development unfolds, let's go back to the earliest days of a child's life. Babies don't start out with a personality; they start life from their core (if immature) self, genetically programmed to be curious, loving, openly themselves and, yes, cautious (it's a big, brand-new, unknown and potentially dangerous world out there), but essentially (in their essence) perfect. As they gradually come to consciousness, babies present their true original self to the world openly. The child cries when it's hungry, and mature, loving parents will respond, in essence: "Oh, darling baby, we understand that you cry when you are hungry. That's the way it should be, and we'll feed you now." The child might then enact another part of its pre-programmed unfolding of self: "I sleep when I'm tired," and the parents might respond, "That's beautiful, little baby. We'll make sure you have a safe place to sleep." Finally, the child enacts a part of its natural behavioral repertoire—say, screaming with rage when a need isn't met—that may not be acceptable to the parent. This characteristic may intersect with a psychological issue the parent has—perhaps it triggers the parent's need for safety and control, perhaps it violates ingrained codes of morality, perhaps the parent had overly demanding parents of her own who got angry at she when they were young, and so she may have developed a personality that is resistant to the demands of others. For whatever reason, this third characteristic of the baby pushes one of the parent's own childhood buttons. So when the child offers this part of itself, instead of responding, "Oh, sweet child, we understand you are exploring your universe, learning about control, and we love you nonetheless (but you still can't have the candy now)," the parent this time says, in essence, "Hold on just a minute there, now, baby. That characteristic will have to change!" (Parents will generally communicate this message through one extreme or the other, either with coolness, by withholding love, or with heat, by expressing anger—emotional "fight or flight"—but either way, it's not centered, balanced, grounded, awake, mature parenting. Either way, it's lacking unconditional love, the primary element of good parenting required by a baby.)

In response to this demand for change, the baby is confused and surprised: "Wait a minute," the baby seems to be saying. "Remember me? The darling baby? You loved characteristic number one. 'That's beautiful, little baby,' you said. And you loved characteristic number two. Now you're telling me that this part of me is unacceptable? I must have heard you wrong. Here's characteristic number three again: 'I scream with rage when my desire isn't met.' Isn't that beautiful, too?" Yet with every action and every emotional nuance, the parents, in essence, say, "No, that characteristic is unacceptable!" and again, the baby's expression of that particular characteristic of its true self is rejected by the parent.

So, what's a baby to do? After trying openly, repeatedly, to be loved, the evolutionary imperative kicks in. There's a fundamental Darwinian survival consideration: the baby is not only frustrated by this treatment, but also helpless and vulnerable. The child doesn't know that there is a world out there beyond the eclipse of the two parents, who are overwhelmingly dominant in the child's ecology. So the baby (in essence, nonverbally, viscerally) "thinks": "Hmm . . . This isn't working. Here they are, two gods in my life, and they are saying I have to change that part of me or they won't love me. And that could prove fatal: if they neglect me I could die of thirst or malnourishment, or from outright acts of violence, if they become enraged by me. OK, I'll switch to Plan

B: personality." The child really has no choice; it's conform or die. That is, on a fundamental level the baby "decides" to conform to the neurotic template the parents are offering it: "Rage is unacceptable. You must be compliant instead." This creates a split between the original, true self and the newly adopted personality strategy that solves the immediate, short-term problem of survival but creates a duality in the baby's sense of self—true self repressed; adopted personality expressed—that results in a lifetime of difficulty, what we refer to as neurosis.

Even so, the human spirit is indomitable and many a child will spend a lifetime struggling to find a way to enable their true self to emerge, despite the over-control or under-love of parents. This is because the true self doesn't go away; it just goes into hiding, in the basement of the organism, with the door shut, locked with many sturdy locks and boarded up with a big sign written in a child's scrawl, saying, "DANGER! Don't go down here! Pain and possible death down here! Stay away!"

Even so, the locked-away component of our true, original self doesn't stay down in the basement quietly. No, it raps on the pipes, bangs on the door, and generally lets itself be heard upstairs in the form of symptoms.

Yet I believe that symptoms are positive—our best friends—in that they offer us the truth, the opportunity to reconnect with our true self, the opportunity to become whole again. So I instruct my clients to follow their symptoms down to the source, to open up the basement door, remove the boards, unlock the locks, and go down there.

When they try to get back to their earliest childhood trauma or deficit ("trauma" from parental anger; "deficit" from parental coldness), they frequently report, in some form: "But there's a monster down there!" and the monster frequently growls out something like, "Go away, or I'll scratch your eyes out!"

In my work as a psychotherapist, the foundation is the development of a trusting, loving, natural relationship with my clients. By the time I advise them to go down to "the basement," that trust should have been established. And so I tell them, "It's not a monster. Try again. Go down there, and this time go toward that voice with love and strength in your heart." When the client tries again, they generally see that it's not a monster but a small child, huddled in the corner, scared and defensive, sobbing softly and saying, "Go away, or I'll scratch your eyes out." Most of us, seeing a little child crying and making such a clearly fear-based, defensive, unconvincing threat, wouldn't turn away, but rather would approach the child (our inner, rejected child), scoop him up in our loving adult arms, and bring him upstairs, set him down at the dining room table with the rest of our personality, and announce to all: "This child, this part of us, was locked away long ago, but is now back upstairs with us, free and entitled to be his true self again."

My clients are able to do this now and weren't as children because, while the pain of receiving immature parenting, of not being unconditionally loved, is still as strong today in our subconscious as it was when it was originally experienced by the young child, the fear of a possibly fatal consequence of the neglect or aggression is gone. This is because while we always need love, as adults we have usually come to feel safe in our own hands. As a small child, we had neither the physical nor the cognitive maturity to survive on our own. Physically, at that stage we didn't have friends or a job; we couldn't drive a car. As a one- or two-year-old, we didn't have the ability to say, "Mom, Dad, you've been providing immature, self-centered, neurotic parenting, and unless you start cherishing my development, keeping me safe, and loving me for who I am, I'm moving out and finding my own apartment!" Ridiculous, of course, in a toddler, but it's just how we might respond were we to experience such treatment as adults.

Furthermore, from a Piagetian developmental perspective, young children simply don't yet have the cognitive maturation to do what we as adults can easily do: take the other person's perspective by putting ourselves in their position, looking at the big picture, thinking of the future. No, a child sees things in black-and-white terms: either I'm wrong or my parents are, this is so scary that I have to bury it forever, and the like. These are the psychological equivalent of that old childhood threat "I'll hold my breath till I turn blue!"—an impossible strategy. Yet by the time the client has become an adult, she is cognitively developed. And once we have created a setting of trust and acceptance, the fear has abated and the basement door is opened, and she can re-experience her childhood fear, recontextualizing it as sad but not overwhelming. She is now capable of releasing that old fear and finally seeing their childhood experience, herself, and her parents with empathy, compassion, and acceptance—with relaxed, loving peace.

So we can see now that personality is not our true self; but rather, it is acquired, secondary, external—strategic. The psycho-logic went like this: "Well, I couldn't get love, approval, and support for my natural trait; maybe I'll get, if not love, at least approval and support—ersatz love—if I adopt this characteristic my parents are so intent on imprinting on me." It's as if the child is malleable clay and the parent—with a "neurotic" personality shell already in place—becomes a mold that is repeatedly imprinted on the impressionable child. Eventually, inexorably, the vulnerable child conforms—or reforms—and personality emerges. It must be noted that the result of this parental press is not always conformity. Often the response to overweening parental pressure is rebellion, even in a young child. Yet rest assured that one way or the other, the child's psychology, the child's personality, will be in play in response to mindless, immature parenting.

With this process specified, we can now see the emergence of a "core-shell" theory of personality development. Our original core characteristics that were not acceptable in childhood aren't eliminated but repressed, and the acceptable traits, both natural and adopted, become the shell with which we interact with the world. That shell is the ego, a natural, adaptive psychological structure that in a healthy individual is a powerful tool used by the self—our true identity—to have an adaptive effect on the world and our survival. In a repressed self, however, out of the fear that we are inadequate, incapable, dangerously flawed, created in us by parental rejection, we defensively place our entire identity into the powerful, effective—safe—ego function. This strategy chosen by our childhood selves is understandable, but a distortion of the healthy function of the ego as tool, not identity.*

Couples Work

In my psychotherapy practice, in particular in my work with couples, I frequently encounter an exquisite, almost eerie sense of balance, fit, reciprocity, duality, and the like. I find that people operate as part of integrated systems, both internal and interpersonal, and that those systems are almost always in balance or homeostasis. For example, if a client is brash in interactions with me, I will immediately speculate that he has have an equal and opposite insecurity, inside as well as outside (often in the form of a projection onto a significant other). Similarly, if a father is harsh, the daughter might be shy, and there is a balance of intensity: very harsh balanced by very shy (or the daughter might respond to her father's extreme harshness with extreme rebelliousness or hostility of her own, but in both scenarios, balance is maintained). Later, when that shy daughter marries a harsh husband in an attempt to complete unfinished business in the father-daughter relationship, we may at first see the harsh

---

*Of course, it is also true that two newborns, side by side, may naturally exhibit very different dispositions. One may be crying and screaming her lungs out, while the second is sleeping soundly right next to her. And these differences persist—longitudinal follow-along research shows that twenty years later, the sleeping infant will have grown into a mellow adult and the crying infant into a more excitable one. This is not a value statement. The mellow adult may be calm and happy or slow and inept at life; the excitable adult may be active and happy or overreactive and miserable. Even so, not all dispositional traits are acceptable to parents, and so personality structures will be crafted in response. It is crucially important to remember that personality is a strategy devised by a baby! Personality is formed during Piaget's preoperational stage of cognitive development—a period of absolutes and opposites, before the child has the capacity to take another's perspective or to think about the big picture or the long term. At that age, we can't mentally rotate objects and we can't walk in another person's shoes. It should come as no surprise that personality—again, a strategy devised at an immature stage in our development—once locked in, ends up getting in the way of one's life, rather than helping us achieve the goals of adulthood.

husband as the one who is out of balance and neurotic, and the shy wife as being more healthy or normal—nicer—but this is not the case. Imago Relationship Therapy describes how in most couples there is a "maximizer" and a "minimizer." The maximizer reacts strongly to every bump in the road and wants to openly discuss all issues; the minimizer takes things in stride and avoids discussing difficult interpersonal topics. Both the maximizer and the minimizer are equally off center, in an unsustainable balance of extremes in their relationship.

Another guide to the health of the system (either within oneself or with the other half of a couple) is the volatility or sharpness of the swings between the two poles of the system. Similar to the chart of stock market prices on a volatile day, some interpersonal fluctuations are sharp, extreme, and unpredictable. On the other hand, when variation around the average is modest, with only a gentle sine curve tracking the interplay of opposites that are in harmony, the system is more likely to be healthy and sustainable. Likewise within an individual, variation between poles of an internal duality can be either extreme or mellow. The mellow variations can be accommodated within one personality, whereas the more violent variations between extremes can't be contained within one personality and require a duality of two separate personalities (such as pushy and insecure) to accommodate. In psychodynamics, there is often a duality between feeling good about oneself and feeling bad about oneself, similar to (and derived from) the duality between the parent's harsh judgment and the child's initial, positive self-image. Once again, these judgments—"I'm OK" but "you're not good enough"—are in balance. In a couple, each person will adopt one of these two subpersonalities: for example, the husband might project "I'm the tough guy!" when in reality, the "tough guy" persona is a false, fear-based, defensive shell. He might likewise project his Other onto his spouse—"she's so weak!" The weak/wimp/loser persona, although equally fear-based, is more submissive and so less reliably protecting and safe, and so our "inner wimp" is often projected onto the spouse so it can be the partner we critcize instead of ourselves.

Imago Relationship Therapy (www.gettingtheloveyouwant.com), ostensibly a couples' therapy, is actually the best all-around tool for *individual* psychotherapy that I've encountered. The reason is that Imago helps us work on the early, formative childhood issues after our parents are too old, or dead, or changed and sweet, or unwilling to talk with us, or any number of other reasons why we literally can't go back. Where does that twenty-four-year-old woman who screwed you up reside now? Not in the more mature sixty-, seventy-, or eighty-year-old woman she's likely become. Rather, our childhood mother is now most alive inside of us, and we can process that relationship introspectively or through our significant other, because in most cases, we've projected our opposite-sex parent onto our spouse and so we've got the perfect symbolic surrogate. Furthermore, it's not that our spouse is just symbolic of our parents—frequently they will actually possess those traits, too. In Imago Relationship Therapy, we are dealing with a real-life, living, breathing person who has many of the traits your parent had when you were young. Distant, smothering, angry—whatever it might be for you.

Why? Why do we choose somebody who has the same limitations that our parent did? Are we masochists? No, of course not. It just isn't good enough to find somebody who is the opposite of our parent, somebody who would give unconditional love. We wouldn't believe it, wouldn't accept it, wouldn't be ready for it. What we need is somebody just like our parent who we finally get to change, who we can finally get to say, "Well, I used to not like you that much, but now I realize who you really are. I should've loved you from the beginning. What a fool I was! But I've changed my mind about you. You're the greatest and from now on, I'll always be there for you." We believe that if only our parent would have said that to us, we would have been psychologically healed! Or, we think now, if only our spouse could be brought to say that, THEN we would be healed! So we keep trying to get that love, never realizing that parental love (or symbolic spousal love) is not the source of our love. Rather, it is the mirror of our own lovability, as seen in the gaze of the mother, that enables us to love ourselves and, that self-love is the true source of self-esteem, not ongoing love from the outside.

A man marries a woman who's like his mother in several key ways and then tries to change her to love him the way he thinks he needs. Of course, the more he tries that, the more he's pushing her buttons and she backs away even more, because, for example, she doesn't like to be controlled—a perfect fit. Psychologically, we pick our Imago opposites who are perfectly awful fits, just like our parents were, and that's how the buttons get pushed back and forth in vicious cycles.

In relationships, there are three broad stages (if we're lucky enough to get to the third phase): (1) infatuation, (2) the power struggle, and (3) a conscious relationship. During infatuation, the partner can do no wrong, whereas during the power struggle, each begins to wonder if they are going to get his or her needs met. Finally, after realizing that a vicious cycle has no end other than when you decide to make an ending, after realizing that the entire power struggle was a massive projection of one's own, one is finally ready to release one's childhood needs and focus on helping oneself and one's partner to feel awake, mindful, present-moment love.

When a couple first comes into my office, it almost always goes like this:

He: Yes, I've screwed up plenty, but she is so incredibly [fill in the blank] that if she would only deal with her problems, my issues would be insignificant.

She: What? It's exactly the opposite. If you would only deal with your issues, mine would be insignificant.

In fact, relationship issues are the issues of an integrated system, of a perfectly awful fit. It's virtually never 90:10, except fleetingly. It's almost always 50:50—or 60:40 or 40:60—but never 90:10, otherwise the relationship wouldn't have lasted for any length of time.

In an Imago Relationship Therapy session you disengage. While the first party's talking, the second party is holding back and listening, mirroring, and validating. Frequently, the partner who's talking will be angry or sad about the other partner, criticizing her mercilessly (the session in my office may be the only time the sharing partner gets to be critical without being interrupted by the spouse, in fact receiving mirroring and validation). At a certain point near the end of this barrage of criticism, I will ask: "Does this remind you of any relationship you had in childhood?" To which the partner who has the floor will often respond: "Yes, it's just the way my moth . . . Oh, shit!" (Or: "Yes, it's just the way my fath . . . Oh, shit!") I call this the Oh, Shit Moment. It is a flash of recognition in the client's mind and heart that he has been projecting onto his partner the anger or sadness or fear he originally felt toward his parent in childhood (and trying to resolve subconsciously through their relationship with his spouse). And this moment is also transformative for the criticized spouse, as she finally realizes that she is not really the source of their spouse's intense feelings and, as they realize that, a remarkable thing happens: she starts to feel empathy for the one who has been criticizing her. Typically, in session, the spouses then switch roles, with the "sender" now the "receiver," and vice versa. During this part of the session, the sender might begin by talking about how it felt to get all that criticism when she was the receiver. Eventually, the question will be asked, "Does this remind you of any relationship you had in childhood?" And so on as both partners awaken from their interconnected nightmare.

The result of the Imago safe mirroring process is recognition in both partners that they have been projecting their childhood issues onto each other. Through disengagement of the typical vicious cycle communications (by the mirroring process and the use of separated sender and receiver sessions), through a developing awareness of one's projections and how they operate, and through the experience of empathy and the resultant desire to help—the very thing each partner wanted in the first place—these couples can now proceed to experience and enjoy the rigors, the ups and downs, and the challenges of a conscious marriage. Finally, a mature, adult, and conscious relationship can begin.

Psychology is the science of opposites, of paradox. If we are scared, we act as if we are fearless; when we try to control, we engender resistance; we hate in others what we secretly hate in ourselves; and so it is with psychological projection. We begin with the neurotic/immature parent interacting with the still-perfect baby. There is some aspect of the baby that is unacceptable to the parent, so now there is an implicit debate: I want this aspect of me (all of me . . .) to be good enough to receive love (the child's position); or, is this trait so bad that expression of it will result in a loss of love (the parental position)? In my clients, this debate is unresolved, is repeated endlessly, and is incorporated into the child's personality, all because the parent's personality has undermined the baby's original confidence in its own abilities.

At this point, the entire debate has been internalized by the child, with the parent's stance now adopted by the child. The debate is no longer: "I want my trait to be good enough to receive love" versus "YOUR trait is not good enough to be loved," but has internalized and generalized to become: "I'm good enough to be loved" versus "I'm not good enough to be loved."

When one meets up with an Imago match, one takes the next step in the process, projecting half of one's internalized dialogue (the negative, painful one) onto the mate. Now it becomes: "My trait is acceptable (and beneath that, I'm good enough to be loved)" versus "Why are *you* criticizing that trait (and beneath that: Why are *you* saying I'm not good enough to be loved?)." The key to resolving this projection is reversing it, and the key to reversing it is to consciously own and then release it. We must first accept that we have been projecting onto our spouse and that the behavior really originates within ourselves. Yet once one realizes that one's debate with one's spouse is just a projection of a debate of self-doubt we are continually conducting inside about ourselves, we not only let our spouse "off the hook," but can also begin to analyze where the self-doubt within us came from. That realization then engenders the final step in the process: recognizing that our internal debate about our self-worth originated in our parent's projection of their negative feelings about themselves onto us and that their projection onto us was an externalization of their own self-doubt. Finally, both sides of the debate about self-worth have been returned to the parents who projected the question onto us (and we can understand, and empathize with, our parents for having had that terrible debate projected onto them from their own parents). Finally we can break the repetitious cycle of projection and pain, passed down through the generations. Finally, we can be fully aware of our own projections and release them through empathy, compassion, and acceptance.

When we awaken to our projections we can dis-identify with the acquired, defensive shell of personality and reidentify with our true core, our original self, through a process of retroactive maturation—rejoining our true psyche in the unfolding of identity that was stunted as a baby. This entails a process of repositioning the locus of our awareness—of self—a process perfected by breakaway Freud disciple Roberto Assagioli, founder of psychosynthesis.

Psychosynthesis

Psychosynthesis attempts to integrate Freudian psychoanalysis with Eastern philosophy. One of the central tenets of psychosynthesis is the concept of the subpersonality. In any five-minute period of any day, we can identify with several distinct clusters of related personality characteristics. Let's say a teen with a new driver's license is driving with his mother in the car, trying his best to drive carefully, when another driver almost hits the car. He might flash into anger, fuming and cursing under his breath. At that point, his mother might admonish him for losing his temper. In the space of that brief period, the young man instantly shifted from the dutiful-citizen subpersonality, to the irate-driver subpersonality, and finally to the guilty-son subpersonality. Assagioli doesn't begrudge us our subpersonalities, only that we are generally unconscious of them. Rather, he would have us disidentify from our subpersonalities and reidentify with our core self—the transpersonal ground at the center of these subpersonalities. Once we are positioned firmly at the core self, we can begin to consciously use and apply the strengths of each subpersonality as needed and in coordination.

Another useful concept to come from psychosynthesis is that of the will. This is not the primitive concept of one person's will dominating another's. Nor is it as simple as the concept of willpower, by which one might exert control over a personal impulse or desire. Rather, the psychosynthesis concept of will refers to the intention of the deepest core part of us. As we release childhood issues and disidentify with personality, when we are in touch with our true underlying self, when we have breathed deeply, relaxed, and released the knots in our psychological "muscle" and are just being ourselves, then our will emerges. Our will is the simplest, most direct expression of our true nature—who we are at our deepest, most relaxed self. At that state of mind, what we really want naturally emerges from our core as the will that psychosynthesis has portrayed. This is not a thinking will. This is the whole, relaxed will that is evoked through meditation.

J. Krishnamurti had a similar perspective on will: that when we have attained clarity of mind or awakening to the distortions in the way we think of ourselves and others, enlightenment is simply the absence of hesitation or encumbrance in the process of being. For Krishnamurti, enlightenment was less something to be attained than it was something to be uncovered or released.

Profile: Swami Allan Ajaya, Ph.D.

Swami Ajaya is a licensed psychologist practicing psychotherapy in Madison, Wisconsin. A native New Yorker, Ajaya still comes back once a month to see patients, and for a time he was my clinical supervisor. Originally named Alan Weinstock, with a doctorate in clinical psychology from the University of California, Berkeley, Ajaya went to India for an extended visit in the 1970s. During his visit, Ajaya met Swami Rama and became his chief disciple and coauthor, later helping him found the Himalaya Institute in America. Ajaya also spent years studying yoga therapy and Vedanta philosophy with various yogis in India. In the West, he has apprenticed and studied with leading innovators of experiential psychotherapy including Carl Whitaker, Ron Kurtz (the developer of Hakomi therapy), Arnold Mindell, and David Grove.

Ajaya has published several influential books, including *Psychotherapy East and West: A Unifying Paradigm,* which takes us from determinism, through humanism and dualism, to monism, a unitary philosophy. His book *Yoga and Psychotherapy: The Evolution of Consciousness* describes the contribution of yoga and meditation to the practice of an integral Western psychotherapy.

One of the most common statements repeated in the West about Eastern philosophy is that the physical world of reality—*maya*—is "an illusion." That's not really so. It's just not all there is, or even the most real or the most important part of reality, but there are few who would argue that the material world doesn't exist in some way, in some form.

Many metaphors apply, but I like to think of the "real" physical world as built on or emanating from a foundation or essence of universal energy—often represented by the word *Om*—underlying everything, a foundation or essence that we call spirit. That energy field is fundamentally different from the structured waves and frequencies that define the cooler, denser, slower, and more stable formats of matter. We can see matter as precipitating out of the underlying energy field much like rain precipitates out of the vapor cloud, as temperature, humidity, and barometric pressure vary.

If one key difference between matter and energy is the frequency, speed, temperature, and density of the energy patterns, then the least-dense energy patterns would be thought, awareness, and consciousness (this is the way reality is conceived of in yoga).

So, rather than thinking of the physical world as all there is or as completely illusory, I prefer to think of the physical world as precipitating out of a more fundamental ground of being. A good metaphor is the mycelium of mushrooms. Mycelium is the true organism, growing underneath the surface; the mushrooms that spring up are simply the individual fruiting bodies of that larger, unseen underground network.

Likewise, we humans are the fruiting bodies of a larger whole of our species, but also of life on Earth—of life in general, of the ecstatic energy field that underlies everything. Yoga says that when we silence the mind, we can hear that human "mycelium," our underlying nature.

My approach is to think of everyone as engaged in a development process. Everyone is at a different stage of that process. The process is what you might call spiritual, but with a small *s*—not Supernatural, but spiritual as in our natural unfolding into maturation, or the development of maturity and wisdom. That is the natural, preprogrammed process we've been genetically wired for through evolution—it's another way of expressing "what works and doesn't get us killed." In the animal kingdom, the plant world, and all around us, individual members of species are in various stages of development through the life cycle. In the case of flowers, they are literally unfolding.

This section has provided an outline of the process of personality development and the dynamics of the baby's own unique underlying self. Once clients begin to release childhood wounds and needs (that until then had directed the contents of their reality), the true self can feel safe to begin to reemerge. I then discussed the nature and development of the underlying consciousness, the foundation on which full mental functioning can be built. It is at this point that clients frequently develop a more relaxed, embracing, and lasting approach to meditation, yoga, diet, and education.

PSYCHE: THE CORE CONCEPT

Who owns the concept of the mind? Is it the believers in spirit, that illusive "thing" that isn't a thing, but somehow resides in the brain . . . or is it the heart? Do scientists own the mind? Those dissectors and understanders who deny something just because they haven't seen it yet? Before Wilhelm Wundt opened the first experimental psychology laboratory in 1879 there was no academic discipline of psychology separate from philosophy and biology. Perhaps it should have stayed like that for a while longer at least: the study of mind from a physiological perspective as a subfield in biology and the study of mind from a conceptual perspective as a subfield of philosophy.

Although there are more psychological issues today that can be significantly and reliably treated by a particular psychological approach than there were one hundred years ago, it remains the case that for most psychological complaints, schools of thought or academic orientation are not related to successful treatment. Rather it is similarity of background and values and the creation of a trusting rapport that are most correlated with successful psychotherapy. Furthermore, for common "neurosis," talk therapy with a skilled practitioner (or even trusted family member) is more effective over the long run than an equivalent-length treatment with any pharmaceutical. Especially since many pharmaceuticals begin to backfire after prolonged use—backfire due to tolerance and side effects, where the benefit begins to be outweighed by the drawbacks. The current tendency to prescribe a pharmaceutical, simply because it works at first, is mistaken. We must find combinations of treatments that are explicitly chosen to be effective without relapse when the chemical is finally withdrawn.

There is an important role played by healing professionals who fight to stop pathology and the damage it incurs. There is also a huge role to be played by those who try to guide healthy, mature living in order to forestall the advent of pathology, especially pathology caused by lifestyle choices, using harm reduction, not moralizing. The psycheology approach I describe next is mostly oriented toward facilitating and guiding healthy maturation and to a lesser extent toward fighting pathology, except during emergency circumstances.

PSYCHEOLOGY:
THE STUDY OF THE SOUL

This book integrates my own evolution into the discussion of using psychedelics for healing. I can illustrate this point by defining a word I've crafted and like to use in my practice: *psycheology*. You won't find the word *psycheology* in any dictionary (I've searched). Rather, it is a made-up word—a neologism (from the Greek: *neo* meaning "new" and *logos* meaning "word" or "statement," or meaningful sound, information as patterned energy). *Psycheology* is a word I created in my effort to reclaim the true, original meaning of the word *psychology*.

The word *psychology* comes from the Greek *psukhe,* meaning "soul," "spirit," "mind," "life," and "breath," combined with the Greek *logos,* here used as "statement," "expression," and "discourse," more often thought of today in the form of "-ology," as "the study of." Although the academic and clinical discipline of psychology has become a medical— and therefore a pathology-oriented—field, prior to the late 1800s, the study of our inner mental life was the study of our soul, our deepest self or essence.

My purpose in writing this book is to bring psychologists, my clients, and us all back to psychology as the study of the psyche, to a focus on the ground of our being, to the soul, because it is this part of us that is the earliest, deepest, and the most authentic part of us. From a psychotherapeutic perspective, the psyche is the part of us that is the most influential in effecting behavioral change and improving self-esteem. Not coincidentally, it is also the part of us that we see illuminated during the psychedelic experience, and it is this illumination of our true nature (or the corresponding "death" of our identification with the ego) that accounts for the therapeutic value of the psychedelic experience. This effect is similar to the concept of sympathetic vibration, wherein a still tuning fork brought into contact with a vibrating one will begin to vibrate at the same frequency. If our conscious attention or identity is brought into contact with or awareness of our deepest ground of being, our conscious awareness elicits or comes into identity with—becomes—

that same deepest sense of self. We are changed—transformed—back into identity with the true self we abandoned in our childhood quest for parental love.

To foster this process of re-identification, we must come to view much of behavior now labeled "neurotic" not as pathological, but as the organism's natural response to developmental and environmental stresses on the path to maturation. From this perspective, "neurosis" is better seen as developmental challenge—the surmounting of which brings maturity or wisdom—rather than as pathology.

The term *neurosis,* as generally applied, is not accurate or helpful. In fact, one of the most negative influences on mental health is the "sick" concept itself, which tightens and distorts, keeping us from a natural unfolding and realignment.

In essence, we need to have psychiatrists (doctors who can prescribe medical and, nowadays usually pharmacological, treatment) treat true biochemically based behavioral disorders, such as obsessive-compulsive disorder and schizophrenia, and return the clinical practice of psychology to the unfolding of the psyche, in all its beauty and complexity, as a nonmedical, natural phenomenon.

With the exception of these biologically based illnesses, psychology must come to be seen as the science of spiritual maturity. We call people neurotic when, in reality, it's not a medical illness they are suffering from, but spiritual immaturity. We must redefine spirituality, too, not as supernatural, but as simply the natural unfolding toward the wise, mature end of the normal curve of human developmental psychology.

In my practice, I find over and over again that big-picture understanding, active listening, and fundamental positive regard work best. From my perspective, "healing" takes place only when we get underneath our modern imago, persona, or personality, to rest at the ground of our being—to naturally unfold according to our perfect, inner template for development. That process both requires and facilitates the emergence of self-acceptance and will.

THE PSYCHOLOGY APPROACH
TO PSYCHOTHERAPY

To summarize, in their approach to clients, therapists with the psycheology worldview will tend to naturally express many approaches from the following list of philosophies and methods:

- ▶ Psychology is about the direct experience of the foundation of our true self. I want to emphasize that in psycheology, we are not talking about the personality but the true, original self—the self we were born as, before our parents "had at us." Our true, original self lies under our personality, in the transpersonal ground of our being, at our core.

- ▶ As newborns, we are all perfect. Of course, we all have individual differences at birth, like the wide-ranging forms of trees in the forest, yet we are all perfect in our essence.

- ▶ Safety—love—is the central issue of infancy; lack thereof results in defensive highjacking of the ego function to create a personality as acquired strategy to attain love.

- ▶ Personality is a strategy devised by an earlier, immature version of our adult self.

- ▶ Neurosis is the natural, stepwise unfolding of human maturation. It's not about pathology, but spiritual immaturity.

- ▶ Empathy and acceptance—love—for our parents and ourselves enable us to relax and release the knot in our psyche, to disidentify with the defensive personality and reidentify with our original, core self—to finally complete our childhood.

- ▶ The desire for change is a reflection of the problem, not of the solution. So, working on yourself or your relationships doesn't work. Rather, the only thing to "do" is simply to be; and simply being is not the result of an active pursuit, but rather the natural result of releasing the self from the encumbrance or distraction of immature personality strategy.

- ▶ Transformative developmental change is possible through a stepwise, dualistic dance—a combination of transcendent and cathartic therapeutic approaches (more on this in chapter 6: The Development of an Integral Clinical Approach).

▸ Psychedelic therapy can be a safe and extremely effective tool in facilitating transformative developmental change by enabling us to see ourselves with love and to safely engage in catharsis. Stunted or skewed development can be gotten back on track, but psychedelics are not cognitive development—or enlightenment—in a pill. Psychedelics can trigger insight, but behavior change takes time, and in this culture, such realignment is often harder to sustain than we acknowledge.

▸ Effective methods exist for changing policies and bureaucracies, and we are honor bound to bravely apply them in the pursuit of science, truth, and freedom (see appendix 1: How to Put Science into Action to Change the World).

The psychology approach to healthy human development is yogic and ayurvedic: seen as a perfect, healthy, developmental process of maturation. Psychology approaches the human organism as a single whole seen sometimes as body, sometimes as mind, sometimes as spirit, but most effectively approached as the integral of all three.

The Beatles had it right: All you do need is love. Love is the central shaping phenomenology of earliest childhood, and love—as essential to life as breathing—continues to shape our existence in fundamental and profound ways our entire life. In infancy, love equals safety, and safety equals survival—we're genetically programmed from birth to seek out love.

Likewise, we are genetically programmed to develop through a sequence of stages that when completed leads to wisdom (or spirituality or maturity). When my son was learning to walk, like most kids, he fell on his butt a lot. After he fell, he would turn to me with a quizzical look on his face, as if to ask, "Is this supposed to happen, Dad?" Of course, I was delighted by all his efforts and would applaud happily in response, as if to say, "Whatever it is you're doing, just keep up the great work!" Of course, I wasn't applauding his falling; I was applauding his trying, his process, because I knew that if I loved his process, he would naturally progress with whatever he was trying. I knew that although he would likely fall again, that eventually his progress would be, "Fall, fall, fall . . . walk!" I apply that same philosophy to the efforts of my psychotherapy clients—I know that it will be, for example, "Failed relationship, failed relationship, failed relationship . . . successful relationship!" So I often find myself smiling deeply when I see my clients struggling; it's not that I'm heartless, it's just that I know where their effort will take them in just a few short weeks, and I'm pleased they are so far down the road.

In his falling while trying to walk and in so many other ways, my son has been my guru. When he was a newborn, I viewed him as an emissary from the land of perfection and found his naive questions profound and helpful. So I have no interest in tightly controlling my son's behavior. As a father, I view myself less as a farmer planting in rows and harvesting output for a purpose, and more as a forest ranger simply keeping a look out for lightning while relishing the wild growth of the natural, unbridled forest.

Another example of being happy in this process is Faith, the two-legged dog. I've always marveled at the difference between the apparent attitude of a human who's lost an arm or a leg and a dog that's lost a leg. As positive as they try to be, the humans are generally at least a little broken by their misfortune. The dogs, on the other hand, are completely unperturbed—they are as joyful and goofy as before. I've often relayed to my clients the sense of wonder I've felt in the presence of a dog missing a leg. Then one day, I saw a cover story in *Animal Wellness* magazine[2] about Faith, the TWO-legged dog (Faith's official website is: www.faiththedog.info). Faith was born with a congenital defect that left her without her two front legs. She was squirming around the shelter on her belly, scheduled to be euthanized, but with an unmistakable smile on her face. A wonderful woman, Jude Stringfellow, and her son, Reuben, adopted Faith, taught her how to stand upright on her two hind legs, and eventually began bringing this remarkable animal into the amputation wards of veterans' hospitals to help cheer up the wounded by exposing them to her remarkable attitude of positivity and love.

I don't believe in neurosis as a pathology—to me, neurosis is the natural unfolding of human maturation. Since everyone is neurotic to some degree or another, it can't be seen as disease. If it was pathological, it would have been selected out of the human population by now; instead, neurosis is ubiquitous. So what could be the adaptive value of neurosis? It is the overcoming of neurotic challenges that brings pleasure, effectiveness, and wisdom.

Is neurosis curable? Yes and no. Imagine the following metaphor: A sapling is growing at the bottom of a hill, when a boulder rolls down, landing right on top of the sapling. The impact is not enough to kill the sapling, however, so over the years, it continues to grow—horizontally, right where the boulder has come to rest, but vertically at the growing tip in the area above where the boulder is. Now imagine it's twenty years later and a kindly farmer sees the boulder on top of the now-mature tree and uses a crowbar to roll the boulder off the tree. Will the tree instantly spring back into verticality? Of course not; that tree has matured and has years of hardened bark keeping it exactly as it was when the boulder was on top of it. The point is that the tree continued to grow toward the light, even with the impediment of a boulder on top of it. While we cannot always change back to our original path after adversity occurs—we can never change our past to be someone who has had fully mature, loving parenting—we can nonetheless find empathy for and accept our adversity with the attitude of Faith the two-legged dog, by flowering and fruiting despite a life-changing event with a psychological boulder.

There is a self-help book with the wonderful title *Working on Yourself Doesn't Work* (and a follow-along book, *Working on Your Relationship Doesn't Work*). The point is that we are naturally, biologically programmed to mature, but sometimes get derailed by our reaction to trauma or a severe deficit in childhood that creates the equivalent of a knot in our psychological "muscle." Knots are treated with warmth and massage, and that is exactly how a knot in one's psychological muscle should be treated, with gentle support and the warmth of loving care. Under safe, loving conditions, we will naturally realign toward the healthful. Even our healing is naturally programmed to unfold, so resist the temptation to help nature along. That would be as if you saw a beautiful red, still-closed rosebud, but decided that you would like to see it open today, and so you get out your tweezers to open up the bud. Of course that wouldn't work and would only destroy a lovely bud that would naturally unfold successfully in its own time.

In my psychotherapy practice, it turns out, paradoxically, that desire for change is a reflection of the problem, not of the solution. Change (in the form of unfolding development) comes about naturally when the whole organism is ready for it; we certainly can't be second-guessing our whole organism, using merely a subset (the rational brain) of the whole. Wanting change reflects poor self-esteem in that healthy self-esteem is accompanied by loving acceptance of the totality of who we are.

One afternoon, my mind was racing around, thinking of all the things I needed to do and trying to decide which of a seemingly endless supply of emergencies I should address first. As I searched my brain for some order or some peace of mind, a phrase came to mind, as clear as if it were whispered in my ear by the voice of an angel: "The thing to do . . . is to be." With all my doing, I needed to simply allow myself to unfold, messy or neat, fast or slow, this direction or that, to relax in the all-rightness of me and my expression of myself.

How do we achieve the level of love and acceptance needed for relaxation, insight, and realignment? For one, through trust in a therapeutic relationship that offers honesty, positive regard, and complete acceptance—a modeling of the parenting clients have missed. Not to substitute for that missing parental love, but to model it for the client to adopt toward themselves. My clients may never have had loving, mature parenting, but they can provide that unconditional positive regard for themselves. In significant ways, my clients learn to parent themselves, to fill the deficit or heal the trauma, to release the unfulfilled needs of childhood. This is why I practice the way I do, developing fond, personal relationships with my clients and responding to e-mails and accepting calls at any hour—because what kind of trusting, accepting, positive presence would I be if I were to defer a client call to a time when we could have a session with a fee? If I am truly optimistic about my clients' potential and delighted with their progress, as I would be with any fellow human being, then I would naturally want to be there with them in their process. Personally, I find it very gratifying. BUT . . .

It is very important to stay aware of and monitor transference and countertransference. As one of my heroes, Sándor Ferenczi, said, in order to work this way you have to be analyzed "to rock bottom"—and that is a daily challenge, but one that I share with my clients and use to further our work. When I fall short of that superlative, it becomes fodder for further analysis of our relationship and so a contribution to the client's (and my own) psychospiritual development.

Finally, I would be remiss if I didn't point out the potential role of psychedelic meditation and psychedelic psychotherapy in the achievement of the kind of grounded, peaceful, happy stability we are exploring here. I believe any mature, sincerely embraced practice would serve to mature us, but psychedelics have the added quality of revealing our true self to ourselves fully, as if for the first time. Seeing through anger, fear, judgment, and defensiveness to our loving, loveable core is a hallmark of a positive psychedelic experience. We will explore this exciting tool more in the next chapter.

3

THE HISTORY OF PSYCHEDELIC RESEARCH

Mescaline was the first of the "classic hallucinogens"* to be widely researched. In fact, mescaline was the original consistent standard by which the strength of other hallucinogens were rated. Mescaline is found in peyote (from the Aztec *peyotl*), which lives throughout the southern United States and northern Mexico, in the San Pedro cactus, native to Peru, as well as in many other cacti globally. Peyote is used ritually and frequently—monthly or more often—in Native American communities, with no sign of abuse or debilitating physiological reactions.

When the Spaniards first came to the Western hemisphere in the 1500s, they tried to suppress the native use of these substances (including *teonanácatl*—"flesh of the gods"—psilocybin-containing mushrooms, another psychedelic visionary plant in widespread use). They succeeded only in driving these practices underground. They are now protected, especially with the emergence of the Native American Church over the past one hundred years or so, which now has a membership of about four hundred thousand Native Americans. A group of Huichol Indians makes a six-hundred-mile trek, round-trip, every autumn to harvest the wild peyote, which is not grown near their home. It is obvious that

---

*I generally use the term *psychedelic* when referring to this class of substance, but bow to common practice and use the term *hallucinogen* when referring to the medical research literature.

peyote is very important—sacred—to Native Americans, especially members of the Native American Church.

Starting in the 1880s, Lewis Lewin, a German toxicologist, received a sample of peyote buttons from the Parke-Davis Pharmaceutical company, which he proceeded to assess. This raises the question of how one does research in the area of psychedelics. Normally when one is testing a drug, one uses animals to test for safety and initial reactions. Yet if you give a lab animal a psychedelic and they stare at the wall, it's hard to tell whether they're having a psychedelic experience. It's also hard to generalize from animal studies to humans. You've got to have human subjects when you're dealing with this sort of substance.

The chemists and the pharmacologists who create these substances are in a very interesting position, because it's pre-research—there are no subjects to give it to yet—and yet they need to isolate the active component. That's done by separating the substance into fractions—layers of its constituent substances produced by centrifugation—and then assaying the different fractions, which means taking a tiny bit. The amount is determined by the typical action of the base substance, but is only an educated guess. Also, it is crucial to account for the effects of tolerance and even cross-tolerance among different types of psychedelics. Every drug has a different tolerance and recovery profile, but with psychedelics, Shulgin's sound practice was to wait close to a week, at least, between experiences. Typically, at the earliest, lowest doses, nothing happens. Over time, by increasing the dose very slowly—titrating—an effect may begin to be felt. At this point, the chemist stops and either convenes a small group to verify his experience or reports these preliminary findings. At this stage, with positive results, grant makers—or pharmaceutical company executives—start authorizing research with larger populations of human subjects (moving first into Phase I trials in a formal research setting to gather safety and dose-response data).

Many of the active researchers in this world have had to be self-experimenters, in the tradition of the nineteenth century, and have exhibited enormous bravery—especially in recent years, when use of these substances has been restricted. Lewin later wrote *Phantastica, Narcotic, and Stimulating Drugs: Their Use and Abuse,* an encyclopedic overview of the range of then-known intoxicants, including peyote. It was Lewin's rival, Arthur Heffter, however, who assayed—on himself—the fractions of peyote, identifying mescaline as the most active component.

Later on, in 1928, Heinrich Klüver published a study of the classic visual effects increased color saturation, geometric forms, jewel-like visions, Oriental carpets, cobwebs, spirals. There were similarities and differences in the visual effects of different psychedelics. With mescaline, colors were enhanced, but forms were also geometric, which is different from the other drugs.

The most notorious psychedelic, of course, is LSD—lysergic acid diethylamide. Albert Hofmann synthesized it in 1938, looking for a variety of actions indicated by the effects of ergot, the classic rye mold lysergide. The familiar LSD was actually LSD-25, the twenty-fifth lysergide Hofmann created and tested in this series. Similar compounds had been found effective for uterine dilation during childbirth, and Hofmann was looking for other useful drugs (some of those drugs such as methergine, which is used to stimulate uterine contractions, are still on the market). With no strong results and animal studies inconclusive, Hofmann formally shelved LSD-25.

Five years later, in 1943, on a hunch, Hofmann decided to synthesize another batch of LSD-25 to experiment with. Apparently, he accidentally ingested a small dose and had what we now know to be a relatively mild, two- or three-hour experience that to him was extraordinary.

Three days later, he decided he was going to systematically re-create that earlier experience to assay the drug's effect. He had deduced that the source of his reaction was his LSD-25, but he knew nothing of the dose he had ingested. To cautiously titrate his earlier experience, he took what he thought was an extremely small dose. In a world where aspirin is effective at 325 milligrams and mescaline at 450 milligrams, so one-quarter of one milligram—250 micrograms*—seemed a very safe place to start his titration. He had no idea at the time that 250 micrograms would turn out to be about six times the just-noticeable dose and almost double the clinical dose. He then had the world's first intentional, significant LSD trip. In fear for his life and sanity, Hofmann made it home on his bicycle—barely. This was on April 19, 1943, and enthusiasts now annually commemorate "Bicycle Day" on April 19th. Four years later, in 1947, the first research paper was published on LSD in the *Swiss Archives of Neurology* by Werner Stoll, a researcher at Sandoz in Basel and son of Hofmann's supervisor Arthur Stoll.[1]

There have been three paradigms psychedelics have gone through over time. At first the researchers saw some extremely bizarre symptoms: subjects were behaving in ways that were comparable, in the eyes of the observers, to the behavior of certain psychoses. They looked at the walls; they saw lights and had visual disturbances; they didn't speak well; they couldn't formulate sentences; they were distracted, made highly unusual connections among ideas, imbued great significance to ordinary objects, and expressed regressive or messianic thoughts about themselves. Sometimes they heard from or conversed with God.

The first explanatory model was naturally called *psychotomimetic*—they thought these substances were creating a "model psychosis" that could be useful in treating, or at the very least helpful in understanding, psychotic patients. If these chemicals could create psychoticlike symptoms in normal individuals, perhaps there is some psychedeliclike chemical at work in the brain of psychotics. Sandoz Laboratories (the current Novartis) distributed LSD widely to psychiatrists who wanted to know what it was like to be psychotic, so they could better understand and treat their patients—a noble idea, but a misunderstanding of the chemical. The CIA funded much of this early research, looking for a mind-control substance to help fight the cold war, under the umbrella of a research program called MK-ULTRA. In the U.S.

---

*A *micro*gram is one-thousandth of a *milli*gram.

Veterans Administration–hospital research, people such as Ken Kesey and Allen Ginsberg were first given psychedelics in CIA-funded studies. Later, each moved on to enact their destinies and the influence they were to project ten years later. In a way, the conservative military of the 1950s was sowing the seeds of its own difficulties (protests, conscientious objectors, desertions) that would surface ten years later during the 1960s.

As early as 1953, psychiatrists were looking at psychedelics as a therapeutic agent—as an adjunct to psychotherapy—mostly to uncover repressed childhood memories. Interestingly, the psychoanalysts, the Freudian analysts in particular, were quick to support this psychedelic therapy. We now know that the therapist's or the researcher's orientation strongly affects the kind of experience people have. So the Freudian therapists heard a lot of childhood memories, repressed fantasies, and the like from their subjects. Jungian analysts working with patients under the influence of LSD didn't get childhood memories so much as archetypes—they got death and rebirth experiences—just as Jungian philosophy would have you think. Likewise, from the psychotomimetic perspective, when the authority figure in the white lab coat comes up and asks, "Are you feeling anxious yet?" subjects would tend to respond, "Well, yeah, I'm going crazy!" This experimenter effect is a strong determinant of outcome and must be controlled for in contemporary research.

One of the clearest findings in psychedelic research is that people are extremely suggestible while having a psychedelic experience. As a result, you have to consider the entire psychotherapeutic field or context—meaning the patient, the environment, the milieu, the orientation of the therapist, and so on—in looking for the effect. Some of the psychedelic experience is clearly placebo effect responding to the enthusiasm of researchers and therapists who are true believers in the cause of psychedelic therapy. It will take years before we understand the basic underlying effect of psychedelics.

Over time, the psychoanalytical work evolved into psycholytic therapy that incorporates moderate-dose psychedelic experiences into ongoing psychotherapy. In Europe, the emphasis is still on psycholytic therapy. Over time however, especially in America and particularly with treatment-resistant cases such as alcoholics, use of a higher dose emerged and came to be known as psychedelic therapy. In psychedelic therapy, the idea was that one overwhelming spiritual experience (or just a few) would transform the life of patients. In important ways, this is still the case with the American clinical approach to psychedelics, in which researchers are finding a positive correlation between attainment of a full mystical experience and changes in the outcome variable (e.g., reduction in substance abuse or end-of-life anxiety).

In 1953, Aldous Huxley was given mescaline by Humphry Osmond, a British researcher working with alcoholics in Saskatchewan, Canada. Huxley wrote the famous early account of that experience, *The Doors of Perception,* which generated enormous popular interest, contributing much to the interest in psychedelics among the general educated public of the '60s.

Soon thereafter, R. C. Zaehner, an Eastern philosophy professor from Oxford, took a small dose of mescaline and had a limited but bad experience. He fought the experience, as the story is told, and then he wrote a book—*Mysticism: Sacred and Profane*—laying out the difference between the real religious experience and the pseudoreligious experience—at best, mere "nature mysticism"—that he felt comes from psychedelic chemicals. Does the psychedelic experience evoke real spirituality or mere "nature mysticism"? Is the mystical experience a physical, biochemical event that can be recreated with a pill or is it something somehow more than our biochemistry? The answer to these dualities is . . . "yes!" That is, the "merely" material world is already, fundamentally imbued with energies and quantum indeterminacies that aren't Newtonian, and the pure-energy world of the spirit is not disembodied after all, but a natural aspect of—grounded in—living organisms (more on this in chapter 5).

Three Types of Neurotransmitters and
Three Types of Psychedelics

There are three major types of psychedelics that correspond to three
of our primary neurotransmitters.

There are acetylcholine "psychedelics"—scopolamine, atropine, and
hyoscyamine, found in plants of the Solanaceae (nightshades) family—
that, as mentioned above, although not meaningfully psychedelic in a
psychospiritual sense, are capable of creating the illusion that an actual
object or person is present, when to the outside observer they are not
(they also create a swooning sense of flying and stimulate the mucosa,
including the vaginal walls). Not surprisingly, these chemicals comprise
the active ingredients in the medieval witches' hexing herbs—henbane,
mandrake root, deadly nightshade (belladonna), hemlock, wolfsbane,
and thornapple (datura). When seen through the lens of "true hallucinogens," stories of witches' brew, flying to a remote coven (on a
broom used for applying ointments), talking with the devil and having
sex with him, begin to become understandable. These chemicals do
carry a heavy "body load"; however, they are difficult for the body to
experience and process. Even so, some kids somewhere in suburbia
are always trying to get high on jimson weed (a form of datura), which,
unfortunately, can be a deadly mistake (and calls our attention to what
can happen when these substances are perceived as illicit and active
distribution of objective information is suppressed).

The second major type is the norepinephrine psychedelics, which
either block, mimic, or enhance the endogenous (internal) norepinephrine system in the body. (Norepinephrine has a stimulating
effect and mediates the body's response to substances such as caffeine, amphetamine, or cocaine.) The norepinephrine psychedelics
known as phenethylamines—for example mescaline and MDMA,
or Ecstasy—are structurally related to methamphetamine and, as a
result, have something of a stimulant action. At high doses, certain
amphetamines are considered hallucinogens.

The third major endogenous neurotransmitter system is the

serotonin system. That's the system that's more influenced by LSD, psilocybin, and the other tryptamines.

Discounting the hexing herbs, then, the two major types of "classic" psychedelics are the phenethylamines, such as MDA and mescaline, and the tryptamines, such as LSD or psilocybin.*

---

*In fact, there is a lot of overlap in these systems, with varying amounts of these three neurotransmitters triggered by any psychedelic. Mescaline, a phenethylamine, does generate cross-tolerance to both LSD and psilocybin (tryptamines). Tolerance has occurred if you take a psychedelic one day and try again the next day and find it ineffective. Either the endogenous neurotransmitter is temporarily depleted, or the number of receptor sites died back, in a natural process called down-regulation that attempts to effect homeostasis in a system that has been overwhelmed by neurotransmitter stimuli. If response to a different class of drug, such as LSD, also shows tolerance after a prior mescaline experience, then the two drugs are said to exhibit cross-tolerance, meaning that the two substances share a chemical and a functional similarity. Not only do they exhibit cross-tolerance, but in clinical studies it's impossible for most subjects to distinguish between the mescaline experience and the LSD experience.

THE MAJOR PSYCHEDELICS

Psilocybe Mushrooms

Psilocybe mushrooms are found all over the world. As mentioned, the ritual use of psychedelic mushrooms was repressed in the New World when the Spaniards came, crushed native use, and sent it underground. Over the centuries, a traditional psilocybin ceremony—called the *velada*—emerged, now combining Christian as well as native aspects. Over the decades, there had been reports of this "magic mushroom." In the early twentieth century, many scholars believed these reports to be completely fanciful, much like accounts of "pixies." There was also speculation that these reports were just accounts of experiences with peyote mistaken for a mushroom (peyote was already well known by then). After an interlude for World War II, it was soon proved that the magic mushroom was real and not just pixie dust.

It was a Morgan banker, Gordon Wasson, an amateur mycophile with a Russian wife, Valentina, a serious mycophile, who finally proved (to the West) the existence of the magic mushroom. The Wassons were rich, they were dilettantes, they were scholarly—and they went to Mexico and, sure enough, did some significant ethnographic research. In 1955, the Wasson team became the first northerners to participate in the *velada*. The expedition spent the night with the soon-to-be-famous Maria Sabina in her small house, hearing her chants until the sun began to seep over the horizon. This was all documented in *Life* magazine, in an article dated May 13, 1957. The Luces, who owned *Life* magazine, were enthusiastic about psychedelics and very well connected, including an influential friendship with the president, Jack Kennedy, and his brothers. It's no surprise that Wasson got a huge *Life* magazine photo spread, and it's no surprise that the Luces' friend, rising psychologist Timothy Leary, read that article and found mushrooms in Mexico. He later developed a complicated relationship with the CIA and the FBI and conducted provocative research at Harvard on the applications of psychedelics.

On a second expedition to Mexico, a colleage came along with the Wassons who, unknown to them, was a CIA agent. Samples of the mushroom were brought back from that second trip to Mexico and were sent to Albert Hofmann, the creator of LSD, at Sandoz Labs in Switzerland. Sure enough, using the assaying-of-fractions method on himself, Hofmann isolated the active ingredients—the psilocybin and its internal metabolite, psilocin,* from *Psilocybe* mushrooms. He also determined how to make it in a laboratory, and Sandoz soon began sending samples to scientists, for cost. They thought this would be a

---

*Psilocybin is transformed in the body into psilocin, the true active substance. Relatively gentle and short-acting—three to five hours—psilocybin is considered by some to have sedating quality to it (one of the first signs of the onset of a psilocybin experience is yawning). It's not surprising that psilocybin is the drug chosen by UCLA, Johns Hopkins, and NYU in their studies with end-of-life anxiety. Statistically speaking, it is associated with the fewest fatalities and the lowest addiction rate of twenty psychoactive substances studied by my favorite mentor, Bob Gable (see chapter 5, figure 5.1).

good way to sell their product, the active ingredient in teonanácatl, the flesh of the gods.

The era of the Harvard Psilocybin Project is perhaps my favorite period, featuring silver-tongued orator Timothy Leary—a bit of an Irish rascal playboy of an academician. There he was, down in Cuernavaca, Mexico, the summer before his new appointment at Harvard, drinking martinis and margaritas at poolside when an academic acquaintance told him that he ought to try the mushrooms. Having read with interest the *Life* magazine article on Gordon Wasson a couple of years before, Leary did. He had a fully wrought, life-changing psychedelic experience and decided, back in 1960, to dedicate his life to the study of these remarkable substances. He was a respected psychologist with a stellar track record in research methodology and survey design. He had a position of enormous potential at Harvard. He had a publication under his belt of a personality test, "The Leary Test," that everybody (including the CIA) was using. He had a book out, *Interpersonal Diagnosis of Personality,* that received rave reviews. Yet as soon as he got back to Harvard, he proceeded to tell everybody who would listen about psilocybin and obtained permission to set up some studies— three of which I'll describe in some detail.

The first study in the Harvard Psilocybin Project was Leary's "remarkable people" study. Basically, they gave psilocybin to everybody, except the undergrads: graduate students, psychologists, religious people, religion professors, mathematicians, chemists, artists, and musicians, in a comfortable setting (usually Leary's house). Results were published in 1963 in *The Journal of Nervous and Mental Disorders,* reporting that 70 percent had a pleasant or ecstatic time; 88 percent learned important insights; 62 percent changed their life for the better; and 90 percent desired to try it again.[2]

LSD

In 1961, Michael Hollingshead and Dr. John Berringsford wrote to Sandoz on Berringsford's letterhead, which was all it took in those days to obtain one gram of LSD—enough for five thousand strong doses.* For ease of handling and administration, Hollingshead mixed his half into a larger substrate, in this case, cake icing, and stored it in a now-infamous mayonnaise jar. Hollingshead showed up at the Harvard Psilocybin Project, and as soon as Leary experienced LSD, the Psilocybin Project turned into, in essence, the LSD Project, because when Leary personally began working with LSD, the gentler psilocybin held no interest for him. Leary never looked back, but I believe the psilocybin study could have continued, been productive, and evolved for many years. LSD is a stronger and a more directive substance, and psilocybin is softer and easier to handle. It's conceivable that there would not have been quite as wild a reaction, or as strong a backlash to the '60s, had the Harvard researchers continued working with the more manageable psilocybin.

Although a stronger psychotropic than other psychedelics, LSD is physiologically nontoxic:[3]

- ▸ There is no chromosome damage from LSD. Other substances—milk, for example—do cause chromosome damage, but not LSD.
- ▸ There is no strychnine in LSD; this is another false rumor. They are similar chemically, but no one has ever found strychnine in any LSD that's been analyzed.
- ▸ Most LSD that you get on the street is very pure, with not too many adulterants. This is mostly because the delivery mechanism for LSD is so small. How much adulterant can you fit onto a little blotter square, physically? The answer, in general, is "not enough."

---

*In addition to Leary, this one gram—referred to as the "magic gram"—also initiated Richard Alpert (who later took the name Ram Dass, meaning "servant of God"), Frank Barron, William Burroughs, Maynard Ferguson, Allen Ginsberg, George Harrison, Paul Krassner, Pete La Roca, Donovan Leitch, John Lennon, Paul McCartney, Ralph Metzner, Charlie Mingus, Roman Polanski, Keith Richards, Huston Smith, Saul Steinberg, Alan Watts, the Yardbirds, and others of the early English rock scene.

Research has found that people with preschizoid personalities—that is, those who are slated to become schizophrenic, often in their midtwenties—on average have a two-year earlier onset of the disease when exposed to psychedelics. Psychedelics are contraindicated for preschizoid personalities and those with a family history of schizophrenia.

MDMA

In 1984, the DEA placed MDMA in Schedule I on an emergency basis. Dozens of therapists petitioned the DEA about MDMA, telling the government that MDMA is not a typical drug of abuse, but rather has important therapeutic medical value. These are empathogens—they engender empathy, so one's defenses don't need to be as strong. With lower defenses, patients can get in touch with deeper subconscious material. This can be particularly useful in couple's therapy. With the use of empathogens, barriers of fear, anger, and resentment are removed, so you can empathize with other people, how they feel, why they've acted as they have, and how they got to be the people they are. Couples therapists in particular found MDMA to be an enormously valuable adjunct to their treatment and were very upset when it was scheduled.

Once MDMA had been placed in Schedule I on an emergency basis, the DEA had their administrative law judge, Francis Young, take a look at all the evidence, including that brought by the therapists. Young took a long time, ultimately producing a ninety-page report finding that MDMA is not a Schedule I drug; it is not even a Schedule II drug, but should properly be a Schedule III drug, available for prescription use in therapeutic settings. The DEA administrator immediately overruled Judge Young's findings. The therapists took the case to court, citing Young's report, and the court agreed: they rescinded the DEA's overruling of the Judge Young report and reverted to the judge's opinion. The DEA refused to cooperate, reinstated its own opinion after all, and in 1986 MDMA was permanently classed as Schedule I.

At raves, (mostly) young people go to a protected space, take MDMA, and dance their hearts out all night, experiencing intense feelings of community. MDMA use has specific downsides—made worse because its illegality limits research, purity and dosage information, and the like. In larger doses, MDMA can affect the length and branching of neurons, and although there has been little definitive data, it's quite possible that long-term use of high doses of MDMA will cause measurable cognitive impairment to memory and perhaps, interestingly, on users' ability to empathize with others (there have been reports of emotional flatness and social indifference in heavy users). There have also been problems with hyperthermia—overheating—and this is simply from lack of information. Kids go to a rave, and they take a pill—or two or three (unfortunately, not having information about the potential for neurotoxicity in multiple doses). They dance like crazy, but don't drink enough fluids, and they get overheated and can die. When information about the importance of maintaining adequate hydration was first promulgated by the community itself, we saw cases of excess hydration—people dying from too much water. Now that good information has been widely disseminated, the problems with over- or underhydration have diminished greatly. The illegality of this substance leads to many problems: poor quality and inaccurate dosing, poor information dissemination, and poor oversight of the management of illegal rave facilities.

In fact, it's arguable that the whole rave scene and the use of psychoactive drugs like MDMA at raves are actually acts of self-medication at the cultural level—youths crying out for a structured, ritualized way to grow, to deconstruct their mental concepts and then reconstruct them at the next developmental level. With psychedelics, we have an opportunity, over time and as a society, to recover a safe and effective way to help ourselves through our rites of passage.

The Serotonin System

Neurons transmit their electrochemical signal through the nervous system across chains of long, slender neurons arrayed end to end. At the end of each nerve in the series, there is a small gap called the synapse. These gaps are linked through the synaptic fluid—they are not actually physically touching the next nerve in the chain. When the electrochemical charge comes to the end of a neuron, it stimulates the release into the synaptic fluid of a chemical that will have a particular geometrical form. This neurotransmitter then floats across the synapse and, fitting like a key in a lock, is taken up by a reciprocally structured receptor site. If there is a physical fit—a structural opening into which this neurotransmitter can fit electrochemically, at the molecular level—then the new nerve cell is stimulated to relay an electrical signal down to (and across) the next synapse. Once the electrical signal has been sent, the neurotransmitter that triggered the second neuron to fire is released from the receptor site and sent back into the synaptic fluid—where, ultimately, it is taken up again by the original neuron, to be reused the next time a signal comes down the neuronal path to trigger its release into the synapse.

This is the system Prozac interacts with as a *selective serotonin reuptake inhibitor* or SSRI. Prozac fits into—and blocks—the reuptake sites in the first neuron where the serotonin is meant to be reabsorbed and reused. When the serotonin is released by the receptor site and it floats back through the synaptic fluid to the first neuron, it finds the reuptake site blocked by the Prozac. As a result, that serotonin bounces back into the synaptic fluid, remaining available and eventually finding its way to the second neuron's receptor site again, stimulating that nerve to fire again. Essentially, Prozac works by keeping more serotonin in play and available to trigger more neuronal firing at serotonin receptor sites.

Psychedelics tend to either mimic or enhance (act as *agonists*) or block or diminsh (act as *antagonists*) the release of neurotransmitters, such as serotonin. If you look at structural drawings of the psychedelics, you'll notice that these substances are structurally quite similar to the neurotransmitters with which they've been associated.

N,N-Dimethyltryptamine (DMT)

Another group of tryptamine psychedelics—DMT (N,N-dimethyltryptamine), DET (N,N-diethyltryptamine), and DPT (N,N-dipropyltryptamine)—is obtained by successive tweaking of the base molecule (replacing the methyl group of DMT with successively higher radicals). DMT comes on in seconds, peaks in minutes, and returns the user back to baseline in a half an hour or so. DET lasts longer—from an hour and a half to two hours. DPT lasts even longer, from two to four hours. As research progresses and we come to better understand these molecules and the way they function in the brain, it will be possible to create substances that result in a very prescribed, specific type of action.

DMT, because of its short-acting nature, has been referred to as the "businessman's trip," because the entire experience can be had and resolved during a lunch hour. Importantly, these substances are not orally active. We have monoamine oxidizers (or MAOs) in our gut that break down substances such as DMT—so unless one takes an MAO inhibitor (MAOI) with DMT, one has to either smoke or inject it. Harmine and harmaline are powerful but reversible (temporary) MAO inhibitors, and plants containing MAOIs (*Banisteriopsis caapi* is commonly used) supply the ingredient that makes the DMT (most often from *Psychotria viridis*) in the ayahuasca admixture orally active.

5-Methoxy-N,N-Dimethyltryptamine (5-MeO-DMT)

Many have been intrigued by the reported practice of "toad licking" for a psychedelic effect. The poor toad in question is *Bufo alvarius* (the Colorado River toad or Sonoran Desert toad), and its skin and venom contains 5-MeO-DMT and bufotenin. Similar to the DMT mentioned above, 5-MeO-DMT (the true active ingredient) isn't active orally without simultaneous ingestion of an MAOI, and so the idea of toad licking is a misnomer. Even so, the skin secretions, when harvested and dried, are smoked for psychedelic effect.

It is interesting to note that toad was also one of the many ingredients of medieval witches' psychoactive brews. One wonders whether eye of newt will eventually be discovered to be psychotropic as well.

Iboga

Iboga is an African root used as a stimulant, aphrodisiac, and rite of passage by followers of the Bwiti religion, mostly in Gabon, Africa. The tribal iboga rite is a very powerful trip that lasts eighteen hours. The ritual is very physically demanding—the participant rages about his personal past, sometimes going into convulsions. It's a very challenging bio-psycho-historical, life-review experience. The active ingredient, ibogaine, has been tested for its ability to interrupt addiction, with brain chemistry and scanning research showing a switch being triggered by the substance in 90 percent of those tested.

THE FIRST RESEARCH ON THE CLINICAL APPLICATIONS OF PSYCHEDELICS

In Leary's Massachusetts Correctional Institution Study, they gave psilocybin two times a week to thirty-six volunteers.* Results showed that six months after parole, the experimental group had a 25 percent recidivism rate, compared with 64 percent for the general prison population.

---

*The word *volunteer* is really difficult to apply in the context of a prison population, and that study certainly would not get approval today, at least not in the form in which it was administered. Why? It is by definition logically impossible for a prisoner to give informed consent completely willingly, as there's always the implication that the subject might get time off for good behavior. Prison subjects, consequently, may try to comply with experimenter expectations or preferences, skewing the results. It's a fundamentally coercive environment: "We completely control your life, and if you do X, then we could do Y, but try not to let that affect your behavior. Just react naturally."

Great results, but twenty-four months later, the difference had disappeared. A later follow-up study by Rick Doblin showed that some of Leary's prison study was falsified.[4]

An early researcher at the Psychiatric Institute of the University of Maryland, H. Aronson also tested LSD response in criminals. Two-thirds were improved in 1963. However, Aronson's group did a follow-up ten years later, and again found disappointing results.

Throughout the first period of psychedelic research (between 1947, when the first human-subjects research was published, and the late 1970s, when the last research at the Maryland Psychiatric Research Center was discontinued), there has always been a strong interest in the effect of psychedelics on substance abuse, in particular alcoholism. This early work was begun in Canada by Humphry Osmond, who coined the word *psychedelic.*[5] The alcoholism studies used predominantly a psychedelic model—high-dose. Because of alcoholics' experience with the psychoactive effects of alcohol, especially delirium tremens, they generally required a higher dose of LSD than what was given for other problems.

In these studies, we see repeatedly that 50 percent or more of the hard-core alcoholics are much improved after six months. Generally speaking, those people who have a profound mystical experience tend to quit alcohol. As William James said in 1902, "The only radical remedy I know for dipsomania [alcoholism] is religiomania."[6] That's still true today.

Bill Wilson, who founded Alcoholics Anonymous (AA), talks in his biography about his experience with LSD. Most people in AA don't know about Wilson's use of psychedics because the philosophy of AA is very different now, but it is true that Wilson claimed that the religious experience he had with LSD was very similar to the religious experience he had that caused him to create AA years before he tried LSD. Once he experienced it, Wilson enthusiastically presented LSD therapy to the AA board as a reliable way to have the life-review experience and spiritual awakening promoted by AA. Unfortunately, by then the negativity associated with the recreational use of psychedelics had already tainted the field, and the AA board emphatically rejected Wilson's proposal.

PSYCHEDELIC RESEARCH IN COUNTRIES BEYOND THE U.S.

In Europe, research with psychedelics was not interrupted as much as in the U.S. In Holland, Jan Bastians, M.D., worked with LSD uninterrupted from 1961 until 1988, when he retired. He found psychedelics particularly effective in people who have experienced trauma, such as survivors of prison camps. In West Germany, Hans Carl Leuner, M.D., used MDMA and later MDMA analogs in psycholytic therapy for many years.

In Switzerland, the Swiss Physicians Association for Psycholytic Therapy was founded, but took a while to initiate good research. Their goal was not research, but therapy to help their patients. The outcome data they did gather found that 85 to 90 percent of their patients considered themselves improved.

In Russia, St. Petersburg psychiatrist Evgeny Krupitsky, M.D., used psychedelic doses of ketamine to treat substance abuse for several years with good effect. Using ketamine, already approved for prescription use, can cut through a lot of bureaucratic red tape.

PSYCHEDELIC RESEARCH FINALLY RESUMES

In 1992, in back-to-back meetings of the National Institute of Drug Abuse (NIDA) and the Food and Drug Administration (FDA), the agencies agreed to allow human-subjects research with psychedelics to begin again. Since that time, Rick Strassman and others have redone the old dose-response studies and now we are at the beginning of a psychedelic renaissance, with clinical research studies underway at several top U.S. medical schools, including at UCLA under Dr. Charles Grob, at Johns Hopkins under Dr. Roland Griffiths, and at NYU under Dr.

Stephen Ross. These latter studies are primarily focused on the use of psychedelics to help the dying, and I give more detail of each in the next section. These new studies are a good start, but far from ideal. There should be clinical research under way at medical schools across the nation (dare we ask for coordination across projects?), there should be government funding available (right now, the government is approving, but not funding, psychedelic research), and there should be a pool of subjects who could benefit from the treatment offered in these studies (the medical establishment is still reticent to refer patients for psychedelic therapy).

THE USE OF PSYCHEDELICS WITH THE DYING

It is significant in the history of psychedelic research that, as of this writing, there are four research projects—at UCLA, Johns Hopkins, NYU, and Harvard University—investigating the ability of psychedelics to ease end-of-life anxiety in cancer patients. While the first research on the use of psychedelics with the dying demonstrated an unanticipated ability to reduce physical pain symptoms (we will cover this research in chapter 5, "Why do Psychedelics Provide Pain Relief for the Dying?"), this section describes the new studies investigating the impact of the psychedelic-triggered mystical experience on end-of-life anxiety.

The UCLA study—"Effects of Psilocybin in Advanced-Stage Cancer Patients With Anxiety," Charles Grob, M.D., principal investigator—is the first psychedelic research with terminally ill patients since the early 1970s. The study examines the use of psilocybin to reduce the psychospiritual anxiety, depression, and physical pain in twelve terminal cancer patients.

The Johns Hopkins study—"Psilocybin and Cancer," Roland R. Griffiths, Ph.D., principal investigator—has forty-four subjects, includes early stage cancer patients, and involves two psilocybin sessions and higher doses of psilocybin than the UCLA study. This research specifically focuses on spiritual experience facilitated by psilocybin as a healing factor in patients who are psychologically distressed by their cancer diagnosis. Outcome measures include assessments of mystical and/or spiritual experience, quality of life, anxiety, depressed mood, attitude about death, use of pain medication, and blood markers of stress and immune function.

The third project, at NYU ("Psilocybin Advanced Cancer Anxiety Study," Stephen Ross, M.D., Principal investigator), is a double-blind, placebo-controlled pilot study of thirty-two subjects to assess the efficacy of psilocybin on psychosocial distress, with the specific primary outcome variable being anxiety associated with advanced cancer. Secondary outcome measures will look at the effect of psilocybin on symptoms of pain perception, depression, existential and/or psychospiritual distress, attitudes toward disease progression, quality of life, and spiritual and/or mystical states of consciousness.

A fourth project, at Harvard under Dr. John H. Halpern ("A Test of MDMA-Assisted Psychotherapy in Subjects with Advanced-Stage Cancer and Cancer-Related Anxiety") is a study of MDMA-assisted psychotherapy in twelve subjects with anxiety as a result of advanced stage cancer, with outcome measures to evaluate anxiety, pain, and quality of life.

The fact that these studies are all under way at prestigious medical schools, with positive findings coming in (as of this printing, none had published yet), bodes well for the reintegration of psychedelics into medical practice. The fact that each of these studies uses the peak or spiritual experience as central to the treatment effect is leading to a redefinition of the role of spirituality in medicine.

THE SAFETY AND EFFICACY OF PSYCHEDELICS

In the West, between 1947 and 1976, there was a phenomenal explosion of interest and research (both inside and outside the laboratory) about psychedelics and their applications. During this time, thousands of peer-reviewed research papers were published in scholarly journals that assessed safety and efficacy and honed clinical practice and research methodology.[7] From a chemical perspective, the classic psychedelics are relatively non-toxic in adults, especially when used in a psychiatric or spiritual setting, especially compared with other drugs of abuse.[8] In fact, the clinical literature agrees that psychedelics are generally, as the old aspirin commercial claimed, "safe and effective when used as directed" (see chapter 4, "The Ten Lessons of Psychedelic Therapy, Rediscovered").

Nonetheless, psychedelics are among the most powerful psychoactive chemicals known and, when used in an improper setting or with conflicted intentions, can cause considerable, although generally transient, psychological distress. When subjects are properly selected and treated, however, the research clearly and repeatedly has shown no long-term deleterious effects from the use of psychedelics under professional supervision.[9] Questions of whether medical or spiritual supervision is most appropriate and when regulated-but-unsupervised use might be acceptable are crucial issues yet to be effectively addressed by policy makers.[10]

I believe there is room for all these approaches—research, psychiatric, ecclesiastical, or shamanic—and others. When used as a medicine, to heal a medical complaint, psychedelic therapy requires medical supervision. When used by spiritual seekers for training, meditation, or psychospiritual development, there is no reason to require more than "on call" medical supervision, even for solo use by the appropriately trained.

These are powerful psychospiritual tools and must be regulated (albeit less stringently than they are now). They should not be available next to the aspirin in the corner pharmacy, but likewise they must not be made unavailable to serious researchers, sincere healing professionals, and mature spiritual seekers. Surely we can craft a thoughtful public policy that would be truly appropriate for these remarkably helpful and powerful tools.

In the next chapter, we will explore whether tribal practices might be a guide to the safe and effective use of psychedelics in modern societies.

4

THE TEN LESSONS OF PSYCHEDELIC THERAPY, REDISCOVERED

Psychedelic plants and derivative compounds and admixtures have been used safely for millennia by indigenous peoples.[1] This tradition of shamanic practices provides the context for the use of psychedelics in psychotherapy and the foundation for our discussion of the methods of psychedelic psychotherapy.*

As tribal society evolved over thousands of years, a set of ritual and community support structures—guidelines of procedure and context—grew up around the use of psychoactive plants. The driving considerations were and are now (1) how to take these substances in such a way that people have the experience that they are looking for and (2) how to do so with the least deleterious effect on the body, mind, and society—the first "safety and efficacy" standards (the key criteria used by modern regulators in approving new drugs). The regulatory and policy debates we're having as a society today may be seen, in part, as an attempt to re-create the controls, guidance, and support that evolved naturally in prehistory.

---

*In this chapter, I present material from a chapter I wrote for the excellent *Psychedelic Medicine,* the first psychedelic psychiatry text book in a generation. (Goldsmith, N. M. "The Ten Lessons of Psychedelic Psychotherapy, Rediscovered." In Winkler, M., and T. Roberts, eds., *Psychedelic Medicine: New Evidence for Hallucinogenic Substances as Treatments.* Vol. 2. New York: Praeger, 2007, 107–41).

Over the past sixty-plus years, Western researchers have systematically reinvented the wheel of ancient practice in roughing out the contours of safe and effective psychedelic therapy. The primary clinical innovations discovered in the West for the use of psychedelics, such as set and setting, turn out to be rediscoveries of methodologies honed through centuries of hard-won tribal trial-and-error experimentation. That being the case, we must now rethink, embrace, and expand upon the tribal foundations, not just of Western practice, but of Western research as well.

What follow, then, are ten "lessons learned" for psychedelic therapy, along with—*in italics*—the tribal foundation for each.

Lesson 1. Each Drug Has a Specific Effect

Match the effect to the purpose. Familiarity with the particular substance, its action, its usual constellation, and its arc of effects are crucial to a successful experience.

All nonordinary states of consciousness are similar, by definition, in that they are different from our consensual reality. Many first-time psychedelic users are surprised, sometimes frightened, by the experience and the realization that states of consciousness other than our default, waking state exist at all.[2]

Plant-based or laboratory-conceived psychoactive chemicals mimic or block the operation of neurotransmitters (chemical messengers in the nervous system that influence perception and mood). The numerous neurotransmitters—serotonin, norepinephrine, dopamine, acetylcholine, and the like—act by triggering or blockading the firing of corresponding receptor sites in our brain. The neurotransmitters fit into the receptor sites like keys into locks. The receptor sites associated with each neurotransmitter come in an array of subtypes. For example, serotonin (5-hydroxytryptamine, or 5-HT) has approximately fourteen receptor site subtypes. To make this even more complex, most psychedelics operate on more than one neurotransmitter system (for example, peyote interacts with the dopamine and serotonin systems, among others).

One way to get one's mind around this complexity is to think of structure-activity relationships—the way neurotransmitters trigger (agonize) or blockade (antagonize) receptor sites—using the metaphor of a large church pipe organ with multiple keyboards. Imagine each keyboard represents a different neurotransmitter system, serotonin on one keyboard, dopamine on the next, and so on. Next, imagine that the white keys represent the release (agonism) of a neurotransmitter and the black keys represent the suppression (antagonism) of a neurotransmitter. Finally, let's think of chords as the complex interweaving of agonism and antagonism of receptor-site subtypes involved with a particular drug's mode of action. Using this model, when a subject experiences LSD, for example, serotonin is the neurotransmitter most heard, but "chords" on the dopamine, norepinephrine, and other keyboards are also played. Furthermore, LSD is likely to play a different chord on the 5-HT keyboard than 5-HT itself (because even at the level of individual receptors, the binding action of LSD is not identical to the binding action of 5-HT), adding yet another level of complexity to the mechanism of action. This rich mix of interactions helps explain how each drug, while based on the same building blocks, will often have dramatically different effects.

Tribal societies have a very purposive and articulated natural psychopharmacopia. Living in an entirely natural environment is like living inside a drug store (and grocery store, and hardware store, and church!). Moreover, tribal knowledge gained over millennia makes living in nature's pharmacy somewhat akin to the pharmacist who has worked in one shop for forty years and doesn't have to think about where each item is kept or even about how to combine them into prescribed admixtures.

For example, the active ingredient in the ayahuasca used in the Amazon, dimethyltryptamine (DMT), most commonly comes from the leaves of Psychotria carthaginensis *or* P. viridis. *However, DMT is not active orally, because it is broken down in the gut by monoamine oxidizer (MAO) enzymes. As such, tribal users long ago learned to add a separate chemical, a monoamine oxidizer inhibiter (MAOI), most com-*

monly harmine from a vine, Banisteriopsis caapi. *Although these are the most commonly used mixtures and all ayahuascas combine some source of DMT (or the closely related 5-MeO-DMT) with some source of an MAOI, there are many different recipes, and the natives have different names for the different types and strengths of ayahuasca.[3] When natives were asked how they came to find this exact combination of active substance and activating substance, among the millions of potential combinations of plant leaves, bark, root, or wood, prepared in any number of boiling, grinding, and filtration preparation methods, and then combined with one or more additional substances with similarly complex arrays of potential selection and preparation, they replied, "The plants told us."[4]*

While this story may be apocryphal, it is clear that native experimental methods have been quite effective. Preagricultural cultures did not have our formal, institutionalized scientific methods, yet experimental designs were used. For example, systematic comparisons must be made among different types of leaves for their ability to be shaped into a drinking vessel, or among different bones for their tensile strength and ability to hold a sharp edge. Without our institutional science, but with generations of time and traditions, a kind of "serial" experimental control would have been used— a systematic, directed trial and error. That is, rather than testing a variety of conditions simultaneously, as we do with experimental treatments and controls, native innovations evolved serially, over time, as prior knowledge was improved upon, trial by trial. This new knowledge was then incorporated into the tribal armamentarium to be maintained and passed down through religious ritual and other, culturally rooted daily behaviors and oral traditions.

Lesson 2. Setting Can Strongly Influence State of Mind and Thus Outcome

Early researchers sometimes strapped subjects to beds in hospital rooms, under the mistaken view that the effects of taking psychedelics mimic psychosis. Most (but not all) subjects under these conditions had hellish experiences, thus seeming to confirm the psychotomimetic hypothesis. However, even in institutional settings, enough subjects had beatific experiences that another explanatory term emerged: *psychedelic,* or mind manifesting. Over the years, researchers and clinicians have generally come to provide a nonthreatening, physically comfortable, pleasing to the senses, safe, and secure environment, often with specific familial items (e.g., pictures, dolls) or religious content (e.g., icons, prayer books).[5] (The setting must be safe and secure not just so there are no outside interruptions, but also to ensure that a frightened or confused subject or patient cannot bolt the session room.)

Psychedelic subjects can be highly suggestible.[6] Although beatific psychedelic experiences were possible in mental hospitals during the early, psychotomimetic period of the late 1940s and early 1950s, therapeutic peak experiences are more readily attained amid a setting with personally meaningful spiritual music and iconography. Far from problematic, this suggestibility is one of the foundations upon which successful psychedelic therapy must be built.[7]

At the opposite extreme, some healing and psychotherapeutic use of psychedelics has employed carefully designed and controlled intensity as a lever to help subjects experience, confront, and resolve their deepest fears and pains.[8] A good tribal example is the Bwiti initiation rite using ibogaine—a three-day, coma and seizure experience that produces a near-death (and sometimes actual death) experience.

The tribal context for psychedelic use is inherently safe. Unlike in industrial society, tribal use of psychedelics takes place in a natural context, both environmentally and culturally. When a young person takes a psychedelic in a tribal setting, it is generally in the context of ritual, frequently a rite of passage from one stage of life into the next, and support by family members and other authority figures is the norm. Later, the entire tribal milieu naturally assists in integrating the experience. No sneaking behind the barn to hide drug use here; rather, this is publicly supported use of a sacrament, in a positive and relaxed environment.

At the opposite extreme, many tribal practices have a fearful and intense component, to stimulate change during the rite of passage. Yet within the supportive tribal environment, these fearful or painful practices are accepted as healing.[9]

Lesson 3. Mind-set Can Scuttle a Beautiful Context or Transcend a Hellish One

Open-mindedness and a willingness to surrender to the process, confidence in the people and surroundings, and a motivation to learn and heal rather than to escape or be entertained, are all associated with a successful outcome.[10]

Mind-set is perhaps the single most important factor in determining the outcome of a psychedelic experience. More influential than setting or dose, set trumps all, because set determines the phenomenology or direct internal experience of those other factors.

Even so, it is difficult to discuss mind-set without simultaneously discussing setting. Setting strongly influences the mind-set of the suggestible psychedelic user, and yet mind-set can overcome the influence of even the most powerful religious or family triggers.[11] Another term, used similarly to *set,* is *intentionality.* If the deepest, truest intent with which one approaches the experience is sincere and one is open to whatever learning is encountered, then a positive experience is more likely. On the other hand, if one's true intent is to avoid certain issues, the stress of that avoidance could cause emotional symptoms that influence the nature and outcome of the psychedelic experience. Of course, such a negative experience is also a developmental challenge, the addressing of which brings maturation and a more open intentionality.

The forces that explain the universe in the animistic worldview are well known by all and are driven by spirits that include the plant aides. The plants are seen as active, conscious agents—plant spirits—rather than as things; they are seen as a means of engaging with the world and with experience that is explicitly reverential.[12]

Tribal participants have completely bought into the concept and practice of using plants for healing and divination and are positive about the benefits to be accrued. Tradition communicates the appropriateness and value of the experience. The tribal worldview fully accommodates the healing action of the ceremonial use of psychoactive plants. Psychedelics increase suggestibility and the sacramental, receptive tribal mind-set is ideal for the effective use of these plants to catalyze spiritual transformation.[13]

Lesson 4. In General, Dose Determines a Mild or Extreme Experience, Although It Can Be Less Important Than Set and Setting

Match of dose to purpose can be crucial.[14] For example, meditative practice tends to employ a very low dose; psycholytic psychotherapy tends to use a small-to-moderate dose repeated over a period of months in the context of ongoing psychotherapy; psychedelic therapy tends to apply one dose or a small number of large doses, aiming for a peak experience; some individuals will use very large doses in their quest for spiritual transformation. In terms of intensity and dose, there seems to be some positive correlation between dose and Masters and Houston's four stages of the psychedelic experience (sensory-perceptual, recollective-analytic, symbolic, and integral; see chapter 5). A mild dose may elicit only rosy colors and a sensitivity to nuance in music; a stronger dose may bring one's focus to psychoanalytical content or a sense of oneness with nature; the most intense doses may bring one to what has been called a "white light" experience, where there is complete dissociation from one's sense of self, body, and surroundings and subjects experience what is referred to as "ego death," a potentially blissful—or terrifying—experience.

With higher doses of psychedelics, sometimes called "overwhelming" doses, the tendency of psychedelics to bring one toward dissociation from one's ego or sense of individuated self is more difficult to resist. At full doses, the attempt to hold back or control the psychedelic experience is costly in emotional stress and almost certain to be a negative influence on the experience of the subject. In some people, at some times, resistance is impossible without regression to infancy, for example, or some other dramatically dissociative temporary psychological strategy for avoiding the anxiety associated with the experience.

While dose can have a powerful effect, mental state—openness and receptivity, mindfulness, and intentionality—can be even more important in determining outcome. Those in a relaxed, open state of mind, eager for a spiritual experience, certainly can have a peak experience on a just-noticeable dose. Of course, such a receptive state of mind can engender a spiritual experience with no drugs at all—and a nondrug-based spiritual experience can be feared and resisted. In fact, some say that our normal state of mind is actually a repressed and impoverished version of the much broader, deeper, and more alive, true and underlying reality experienced by yogis and physicists that, in our immaturity, we resist.[15]

There is a difference of opinion on whether ramping up to full dosage over a number of experiences reduces the potential for panic or simply enables the subject to develop, maintain, and incrementally increase defenses. Generally, smaller doses are used for ongoing psychotherapy, larger doses for transformative practice. The psychedelytic approach combines these two, alternating periodic large doses with ongoing smaller doses.[16]

Tribal practices are specific as to the recommended doses for purposes such as hunting, healing, or divination. The native dose has frequently been described as large—overwhelming—by many Westerners. Yet the full integration of sacred plants into the tribal worldview and lifestyle means that these substances are woven into the day-to-day lives of natives. An example is Huichol mothers providing doses of mescaline as they nurse their infants or biting off small pieces of peyote buttons to feed to their babies.[17] This usage by children, in the tribal context, has resulted in no negative neurochemical or developmental consequences.[18]

Lesson 5. Preparation and Knowledge Can Enable Lasting Value

If the psychedelic experience is a "trip," then, as with any journey, it must be prepared for in advance. Mental and physical preparations in the days before the experience are associated with a beneficial outcome.

An attitude of open acceptance toward oneself and the upcoming psychedelic experience is important, as is familiarization of the subject with writings on the experience he or she is about to have. The subject or patient should be in touch with his or her own inner issues, through psychotherapy or a spiritual practice.[19]

It is wise to eat digestively undemanding foods the prior day or two (avoiding spicy foods, meat, salt, alcohol, caffeine) and to have an empty stomach for the experience itself. Furthermore, planning for a day out of contact with friends, family, and colleagues and preparing a setting with no interruptions are important to a relaxed, focused experience.

Relatives and shamans focus the tribal participant on the problem, illness, object lost, mate's infidelity, or other issue prior to the medicine work. Yet through their upbringing, their shamans, and their own experience with ritual, tribal participants are fully familiar with the expected effects of their ecosystem's sacramental plants. Participants are generally accepting of the process—that the spirits, while not completely predictable, are subject to sincere entreaty. Thus the tribal user enters into the psychedelic experience knowledgeable, optimistic, accepting, and willing. While the content seen or outcome of the encounter with the sacred plant is unpredictable, the nature of the experience itself is not a surprise at all, fitting in as it does so fully into the native culture and perspective.[20]

Lesson 6. Ritual Can Transmit Prior Wisdom and Guide Successful Practice

The UDV ayahuasca churches are good examples of a modern approach to psychedelic ritual in a churchlike setting; another example is the Native American Church and their prayer service using peyote as sacrament. All three accepted, legally sanctioned churches are modern, syncretic creations combining elements of Christianity with elements of the native pantheon of spirits and tribal ritual. In creating such a vehicle, these churches have borrowed perennial truths and religious elements—in whole or in part—chosen rituals, and developed symbologies and ways of interpreting spiritual experiences that reflect, preserve, and transmit their values and successful practices.[21]

Over the decades of modern research, the psychedelic community has learned to benefit from the accumulated wisdom of previous practitioners—for example, to have procedures, guidelines, logistics, set and setting, and security in place.[22] In a sense, methodological protocols and guidelines for successful clinical practice ARE our modern-day rituals—practices honored for their effectiveness in producing specific states or outcomes, repeated over generations, with only slow accretion of newly accepted innovations. The use of standardized practices (rituals) in psychedelic therapy provides a way to inculcate dramatically, to imprint, safe and effective methods. When we require careful preparation, support, a positive set and setting, follow-up, and the like, we are engaging in ritualized behaviors that reflect, preserve, and transmit our values and successful practices.

Today, ritual in psychedelic therapy can offer an outlet for needs formerly met by highly organized, highly ritualized religions, such as shamanic practices or traditional Catholicism. Yet we must remain flexible, as some individuals may not respond well to ritual. Even so, metaprotocols for specific types of needs, such as for church study groups, substance abusers, teenagers, newlyweds, and the dying may provide valid and reliable procedural anchors with which to successfully bring psychedelic practice to the general population.[23]

Tribal rituals instantiate the trial-and-error discoveries of ancestors. Western science uses laboratory controls to compare multiple treatments simultaneously (call it "horizontal" research design), while tribal comparisons of multiple practices occur over millennia of experimentation (vertical design). Nonetheless, the results of tribal experimentation over time concur with—and indeed can guide in their contextual wisdom—results only now being seen in Western research.

Rituals organize rites of passage, helping the community navigate the individual or age cohort from one stage of life to another.[24] *Rite-of-passage rituals symbolize and transmit time-honored truths about the nature of each stage in life and the mind-sets and practices most likely to facilitate successful transition.*

On the other hand, tribal ritualized practices tend to be more formal and deterministic than much of Western psychotherapeutic practice (if not Western religious practice). In part to address this perceived rigidity, scholars at the Council on Spiritual Practices in San Francisco are attempting to create a modern psychedelic religious ritual that is profoundly meaningful, but not dogmatic.[25]

Lesson 7. Support from Experienced Guides Reduces Fear and Increases Benefit

We have learned to involve trusted significant others—family, therapist, physician—in the process of psychedelic therapy. In most contemporary models, significant others communicate with the subject before, are nearby during, and are available after a psychedelic treatment. The focus is on the benefit to the participant, and guidance is responsive to request, rather than proactive or directive.[26]

There is some debate as to the wisdom of having a psychedelic experience alone. Clearly, psychotherapy would not be taking place during a solo psychedelic experience. However, profound meditation and introspection generally results, and the content of the session could produce significant fodder for subsequent therapeutic discussion and analysis. Even if the choice is made by an experienced adult to have a solitary experience, supportive others should be readily available.

One way to mix solitary with supported experience is to have a group experience with places available for solo exploration. Another way to mirror tribal experience is to include a range of age groups, from young adults to elders.

In tribal practice, depending on the culture and the purpose, a psychedelic experience may entail the shaman being the only one who takes a psychedelic, the tribal participant and the shaman ingesting the psyche-delic together, a rite of passage or other group ritual, or the entire tribe participating.[27]

In tribal ritual, the whole family can be involved! In addition to the doctor-therapist-pharmacist-priest (that is, the shaman) and the mayor-police chief (that is, the tribal chieftain), the immediate and extended family may be present. When difficult developmental chal-lenges growing out of a psychedelic ritual are experienced, then or later, they occur with the full knowledge and support of experienced, loving role models. If a youth experienced a difficult time at a rite of passage and was grappling with the transition, he or she wouldn't have to hide, but could count on any number of clanmates able to discuss the issues being experienced.

Lesson 8. Reentry in to a Supportive Community Context Aids Retention

Many epiphanies are lost and resolutions broken by the "after-the-marathon-weekend" effect—that is, reentry into the same context in which the problem was developed. To maintain benefits, it is best for a patient's life context to be supportive and proactive (not illicit and secretive) toward psychedelic therapy. This is one of the reasons why the hippies of the 1960s decided to "get back to the land" and create remote, self-sustaining communes.[28] Even so, every bodhisattva must return to society until all are liberated, and to derive full, healthful, integral benefit from psychedelic experiences, engagement in consensus reality must be seen as part of the good work of personal and societal development.

Supportive online communities are increasingly important, espe-cially as such support is so sparse in the physical world in today's pre-dominantly conservative cultural and political environment. However, online communities and a few pockets of tolerance in urban centers do not provide a substitute for the interwoven hearts, minds, and eyes of tribal members. The implication being the necessity for fundamental sociocultural change (see Appendix 1: How to Put Science into Action to Change the World).

The tribal system is an excellent example of a unified, supportive community context (one actively acknowledged and emulated by the hippies). The tribal worldview is completely consonant with the experience of psychedelics. The nonstandard nature of the psychedelic experience is accepted and readily explainable within the standard philosophies and perceptual, cognitive, and conceptual expectations of animist cultures.[29]

Lesson 9. Accompanying Depth Psychotherapy (If Needed) and Ongoing Spiritual Practice Offer the Main Opportunity for Lasting Growth

Since psychedelics generally don't effect "cures," gains in psychological peace and spiritual maturity must be maintained with the support of an ongoing practice. For certain needs or areas of focus, this practice might be psychotherapy; for others, spiritual practices such as yoga, meditation, chanting, and prayer might be employed.[30] Adopting a course of psychotherapy or spiritual practice is both an aid to and a sign of change,[31] and the associated psychospiritual worldview that emerges has been correlated with improved and maintained health.[32]

Huston Smith warned us that a spiritual experience is not the same thing as a spiritual life.[33] Aldous Huxley referred to the psychedelic experience as a "gratuitous grace," in that it was not predictable, deserved, or attainable through effort. Rather, it was a state of grace without reasons why or strings attached.[34] Yet a spiritual experience induced out of context of the rest of one's life and history is like a cut flower: beautiful, but with no prepared foundation in which to root and grow, doomed to fade.

Spiritual practices are already a deep part of tribal life, before, during, and after a psychedelic rite, and so new development is readily integrated into a preexisting fabric of self-in-culture-in-nature.

Lesson 10. A Revised Worldview Is Both a Requirement for and a Result of Integrated Psychedelic Practice

An integral* worldview integrates mind and body, energy and matter, spirit and the material world that precipitates out of it. This neo-animist perspective accepts and reinterprets such disparate phenomena as emergent properties, synchronicity, extrasensory perception, health, chi, and spirituality into a view of the universe as fundamentally alive and minded.[35]

How does this worldview facilitate—and result from—psychedelic healing? The very question implies the prior question of what it is that is being healed—our psyches, our relationships and families, our nation, our politics and history? Further, in an integral, post-postmodern world, what is actually doing the healing? Medicine? Drugs? Therapy? Spiritual practice? Compassion? Service? Love? What perspectives and methods have emerged over time as consistently effective,[36] and what would such a "perennial" treatment look like?[37] Finally, what would be a reasonable action path to a future with a healing worldview, a worldview that is transcendent but not apathetic?[38]

---

*I am defining *integral* broadly, as the fifth of five successive worldviews. The first worldview is *tribalism,* with an animistic view of a living and symbolic environment. The next worldview is *agricultural,* characterized by dominance and hierarchies. The third worldview, *modernity,* applies a mechanistic model of an inanimate, "billiard-ball" environment, populated by individual people and objects who have inherited the physical world from those in prior generations who subdued it. The fourth worldview, *postmodernism,* takes that billiard-ball worldview and deconstructs it—existentially free from millennia of baggage on which modernity rides, the postmodern worldview disintermediates history from the process of living, enabling the postmodern citizen to live his or her own life. The fifth worldview and the one into which we are developing, the *integral,* reanimates the world, but having been through postmodernity, does so without the use of symbolic gods and spirits, fully cognizant of the mechanistic substrate. This holistic integration of the mechanistic and the animistic—and transcendence of the dualism of their opposition—characterizes the integral worldview as we define it for the purposes of this chapter.

We in the West are coming around, full circle, to a neo-animistic worldview. Tribal cultures exist in a world seen not only as alive, but also as spiritual in essence, by nature. The universe, and the people within it, are seen as magical, but not supernatural. This post-postmodern Western view that integrates mind, body, and spirit both reflects and distills the tribal worldview.[39]

~~~

While we want to benefit from the tribal perspective, we must not idealize it. Both the tribal and integral worldviews share a unitary philosophy, yet they are distinguished by more than simply differing degrees of organization and technology. There is a difference between the simple unitary view that the environment and self are all part of an underlying, unifying energy, and the more complex experiential unification and integration of previously disparate—sometimes diametrically opposite—elements of a greater whole.[40] The tribal perspective accommodates the material and the spiritual by never splitting the two in the first place. The material world is seen as a fundamentally spiritual place. The integral perspective accommodates the material and the spiritual, already split by modernity, by reuniting them through a transcendence of their duality—an integral perspective, not just a unitary one.

5

MANY THORNY THEORETICAL AND METHODOLOGICAL QUESTIONS REMAIN

Clearly, psychedelics have potential for use in psychiatric research and practice,[1] and in 1992, the FDA resumed approving human-subject research with psychedelics.[2] Nonetheless, there are still many methodological and theoretical questions left unanswered. These include the following particularly difficult questions:

- ▸ Why does psychedelic research require self-experimentation?
- ▸ How will we train a new generation of psychedelic researchers and therapists?
- ▸ Why redo psychedelic research already conducted in the '50s and '60s?
- ▸ How should psychedelics be rescheduled?
- ▸ Why do psychedelics give pain relief?
- ▸ Can psychedelics provide lasting change?
- ▸ Can psychedelics induce real spirituality?

WHY DOES PSYCHEDELIC RESEARCH REQUIRE SELF-EXPERIMENTATION?

When Western science began focusing on these substances, the first model of research was ethnographic. This was the age of European exploration and colonization, which was largely characterized by repression of these substances, although some early naturalists and clergy did make note of the practices of the natives. By the late nineteenth century, some began gathering samples and bringing them back to fractionalize (separate into component compounds), assay (identify the components), and titrate (try small amounts of the fractions to characterize the effects of each). In this way the second phase, that of self-experimentation, began.[3]

There has always been a strong element of bravery involved in the history of psychedelic research. The concept of assaying by pharmacologists—in their labs, on their own—has fallen very much out of favor in the scholarly community these days and must come to be accepted again in research with psychedelics.[4] In addition, it is not just self-experimentation, but human-subjects experimentation, more generally, that is integral to this history and is essential to consider in designing policy for psychedelic research. While there are markers of psychedelic effects in laboratory animals (e.g., excessive grooming behavior), such measures will always be inferential. To test the higher-order effects of psychedelics, we must use human subjects. Finally, giving these substances to subjects in safe, non-laboratory settings (to facilitate positive, appropriate mind-sets) can also be important. All of which leads to the conclusion that while regulating psychedelics is appropriate, restrictive control of research scientists is not.[5]

There are enormous issues of personal freedom for the patients as well; for example, if a patient is dying and simply wants an ego death–rebirth experience to ease the process.[6] The psychedelic treatment would not influence the outcome of his or her physical illness, but it could provide very important psychological benefits. Can we ethically deny a dying patient the freedom to direct his or her treatment?

Moving even further out into the public arena, the next question becomes: What about people who don't want a psychedelic experience for any clinical or therapeutic reason, but just for what they view as a spiritual experience?[7] At the end of the spectrum of practice, what about those who are interested only in nonmedical, nonspiritual, "recreational" use? How much risk, public resources, and information dissemination are we prepared to implement—and pay for—to accommodate recreational use? These are some of the value judgments that we as a society are obliged to make.

HOW WILL WE TRAIN A NEW GENERATION OF PSYCHEDELIC RESEARCHERS AND THERAPISTS?

Related to the questions above is how we will train our psychedelic researchers and future psychedelic therapists. According to R. Gordon Wasson: "We are all divided into classes: those who have taken the mushroom and are disqualified by our subjective experience and those who have not taken the mushroom and are disqualified by their total ignorance of the subject."[8] How can we possibly expect someone who has not had the psychedelic experience to be able to facilitate a research project or help a psychotherapy patient in the throes of such an intense and unique experience? So how will we train our psychedelic researchers and therapists? Actively—that is, by having the psychedelic experience themselves in the professional, safe context of a beautiful clinical setting, tried and honed by the sitters, monitors, and facilitators trained for this research. In fact, there is already an approved research protocol for doing exactly that. Here is the section from the proposal to the FDA that relates to training the "study monitors" with an active dose of MDMA:

A second purpose is to provide legal opportunities for so-inclined therapists in our training program to gain valuable professional experience that we believe may help us improve participant outcomes in terms of both safety and efficacy.

In the long run, should MDMA ever become a prescription medicine, FDA is likely to require physicians to complete certain training programs before they can prescribe MDMA. How these training programs should be structured, and whether they may include the opportunity to volunteer for an MDMA-assisted psychotherapy session, are questions that we beginning to address in this protocol and in our therapist training program.

At present, there are no parallels to this situation because there are no psychoanalytic agents that therapists administer acutely to patients to enhance the psychotherapeutic process. However, personal therapy and the experiencing of one or more elements of psychotherapy while in training to become a psychotherapist has been and continues to be a common practice in training to be a psychotherapist. For example, psychiatrists who seek to become psychoanalysts must first go through their own psychoanalysis. Practitioners of Eye Movement Desensitization and Reprocessing (EMDR) for the treatment of PTSD undergo EMDR themselves during their training. It is because MDMA is a controlled substance that our training program needs to involve an FDA-cleared and IRB-approved protocol in order to provide an analogous experience for our trainees.

All four of the therapists conducting MAPS' Phase 2 MDMA/PTSD pilot studies who have had prior personal experience with MDMA in a therapeutic setting before MDMA was criminalized (Dr. Michael Mithoefer, Annie Mithoefer, BSN, Swiss psychiatrist Dr. Peter Oehen, Swiss psychologist Verena Widmer) believe their subjective experience with MDMA has helped them to become more effective in administering MDMA-assisted psychotherapy to their subjects. The two co-therapists who will soon start our Canadian MDMA/PTSD (approved by Health Canada and IRB Services), Canadian psychiatrist Dr. Ingrid Pacey and Canadian psychologist Andrew Feldmar, MA) have also had prior experience with MDMA in a therapeutic setting before MDMA was criminalized. They believe they will be more effective in administering MDMA to subjects as a result of their prior experience with MDMA in a therapeutic context.

Virtually all the pioneering psychiatrists and psychologists who conducted LSD research are of the opinion that self-experience with LSD enhanced their ability to administer LSD within a clinical context.

There is a precedent in the history of the Food and Drug Administration (FDA) for the administration of MDMA in the context of a training program. In the 1970s, in the "Training Project for Mental Health Professionals" conducted at the Maryland Psychiatric Research Center under Dr. Albert Kurland's IND for d-lysergic acid diethylamide (LSD), 108 people with pastoral and counseling jobs were permitted by the FDA to receive LSD up to three times in a therapeutic context. The purpose of the program was to help the mental health professionals to better understand the LSD experience so as to enhance their ability to work with people who discussed LSD experiences with them.

William Richards, Ph.D., a therapist who administered the LSD to many of these mental health professionals, has written a description of the program for our submission of this protocol to the FDA. He reports in his letter, included in this submission, that "in those days, all clinical employees at the Maryland Psychiatric Research Center (psychiatrists, psychologists, psychiatric nurses) involved in interactions with human subjects during the period of psychedelic effects participated in a similar training program as part of their on-the-job training when they first were hired." Daniel Helminiak, a therapist who participated in this program, believed that he benefited as a therapist from undergoing experience with LSD, as he expressed in a letter submitted to the FDA in support of this protocol and included along with this response.

Currently Richards is working as a therapist on research at Johns Hopkins being conducted by Principal Investigator (PI) Roland Griffiths, Ph.D., investigating whether psilocybin can generate mystical experiences (Griffiths et al., 2008; Griffiths et al., 2006). Richards is also a therapist on a second study at Johns Hopkins examining the role of psilocybin-assisted psychotherapy in treating cancer patients with anxiety. He is the most experienced psychedelic psychotherapist and researcher still working in the field, and his views on the value of subjective experience in the training of the therapist carry considerable weight.

In association with lead author, Matthew Johnson Ph.D., William Richards and Roland Griffiths have recently published an article in the Journal of Psychopharmacology, entitled, "Human Hallucinogen Research: Guidelines for Safety" (Johnson et al. 2008). . . . They discuss the desired qualities and training of the research team members who they call "study monitors," who are present with the patient during his or her psychedelic experience. MAPS calls these people "co-therapists." They write, "Monitors should have significant human relation skills and be familiar with descriptions of altered states of consciousness induced by hallucinogens. Personal experience with techniques such as meditation, yoga, or breathing exercises may also prove to be helpful in facilitating empathy for volunteers that experience altered states of consciousness during hallucinogen action." [underline added]. In their attached letter, prepared for submission to [the IRB] in support of this protocol, they go on to say, "Although not specifically stated in the above quote or elsewhere in our manuscript, we believe that, if conducted in a safe and legal clinical context as proposed in your protocol, administering the hallucinogenic compound (e.g., MDMA in your study) to the therapists/monitors as part of their training is likely an optimal approach for helping therapists/monitors understand the subjective effects of the compound and therefore to facilitate empathy for volunteer/patient experiences."[9]

With the current spate of clinical research producing positive results and dozens of new "study monitors" or cotherapists being trained (many of whom are psychiatric residents), we will need to use the best means available to create a new generation of effective, empathic professionals. Training therapists with an active dose of the substance they will be administering to study subjects and ultimately to patients is clearly the most effective process available and should become the standard for such training.

WHY REDO PSYCHEDELIC RESEARCH ALREADY CONDUCTED IN THE '50S AND '60S?

Research methodology and ethics have changed considerably since psychedelic research was in full swing forty or fifty years ago.[10] Methodologically, we have become more sophisticated about and thus more sensitive to the subtler threats to the validity of our research. Such threats include selection bias (due to improper sampling techniques), the demand effects of the authority figure in the white lab coat, and the differential effect of the greater attention given the experimental group, all of which can subliminally influence results and limit our ability to generalize from the data.[11]

For much of modern psychedelic research in the early period (1947–1976), control groups were infrequently used, random assignment to experimental groups was rare, and outcome measures were inconsistent across studies. Furthermore, in those studies with a control group, TLC (tender loving care) and post-treatment follow-up, when included in the study, were frequently provided only or preferentially to the experimental subjects. This methodology calls into question the validity of inferences drawn from the data.

For example, if the treated subjects had a shared experience with the researchers, they could have developed more of a sense of belonging and acceptance. If, due to the special attention, the experimental subjects developed more positive feelings than the controls, they could have been more likely to feel like staying in the program. There could be more subjects to follow up on among the experimental group than would be expected by chance, thus skewing the results. It can be a wonderful experience to feel so cared for, and that component could provide a potential rival hypothesis to explain any salutary effects observed.

Then again, it might not, but we cannot tell from the studies, because many were not designed to control for that influence. We must conclude that in many of the early studies, due to the research design there tend to be significant threats to the validity of the assumption that the psychedelic treatment was responsible for the positive effects observed.[12]

There are alternatives to double-blind (where neither the subjects nor the researchers know who received the active treatment and who received the placebo), randomized control-group research designs; for example, using the subjects that receive the active substance as their own control group—that is, by giving them an active placebo usually prior to the psychedelic session. Nonetheless, double-blind, randomized control-group research designs are the "gold standard" of contemporary research for the many good reasons I outlined above (such as the TLC effect and other threats to the validity of the airtight logic of research conclusions).

It is important to acknowledge that many in the psychedelic research community have always assumed that since the psychedelic effect is so powerful, placebo studies were a sham—that as soon as the psychedelic treatment comes on, everyone will know who received the psychedelic and who received the placebo. While this has often been the case, if the placebo is chosen carefully to be active (if not psychoactive), then placebos can indeed fool the subjects as well as objective observers a significant amount of the time. In the recent work with psilocybin at Johns Hopkins, for example, the (very experienced) primary study monitor or sitter was fooled by the active placebo (methylphenidate, or Ritalin) approximately 20 percent of the time. That is still less than would occur simply by chance (50 percent of the time) if no difference was being detected, but especially if we consider that some of the 80 percent-plus correct assessments were not certain. This does indicate that placebo-controlled studies are not worthless and that further efforts may be able to develop improved placebos (or combinations of substances as a placebo).

HOW SHOULD PSYCHEDELICS BE RESCHEDULED?

Since the current clinical research programs with psychedelics are finding good to excellent results, and since we are in the process of training dozens of new psychedelic researchers, many of whom will want to become psychedelic clinicians, the trend lines are clearly pointing to—begging for—the rescheduling of psychedelics (in particular, psilocybin and MDMA). What follows is a discussion of the scheduling process and criteria and how psychedelics fit into that system and the likely outcome of efforts to reschedule psychedelics.

At the broadest level the government's scheduling criteria are based on safety and efficacy (although it gets much more fine-grained than that, as I will discuss below). In terms of safety, we can begin with the animist or tribal tradition, wherein these substances—in the form of visionary plants—have been used safely for millennia. Through a process of trial and error, tribal peoples learned what worked and what didn't and incorporated successful practices into ritual that was passed down from generation to generation, with improvements made incrementally over time.

In modern times, Western civilization, with its extractive, reductionist power orientation, has isolated the active ingredients of the tribal visionary plants. While plants such as opium can produce highly addictive substances such as morphine and heroin (and fermented grape wine can be distilled into 86-proof spirits), the active ingredients of visionary plants tend to be nontoxic chemically, although they may be psychospiritually overwhelming or even dangerous. For example, while LSD is active in microgram doses, the LD50 dose (the amount that will kill 50 percent of the experimental animals) has never been established. In addition, psychedelics are meant to be taken in one or a few acute administrations (or, in psycholytic psychotherapy, in lower doses over a period of months, but with administrations separated by one or more weeks). Most psychiatric pharmaceuticals, on the other hand, are meant to be taken in chronic daily use, often for a lifetime. Finally, although the effects of psychedelics are powerful, they are transient and this includes even the most difficult experiences (when contraindicated circumstances, such as a family history of schizophrenia or bipolar disorder are pre-screened out).

The efficacy of psychedelics has likewise been demonstrated over millennia of tribal use and, more recently, in Western clinical research studies (and in clinical practice before they were criminalized in the 1960s and 1970s), demonstrating at the very least strongly suggestive medical uses in a myriad of application areas including:

- creativity
- criminal recidivism? (The question mark reflects the flawed methodology of the research that attempted to demonstrate this application.)
- cluster headaches
- substance abuse and addiction, especially alcoholism
- relationship counseling
- childhood autism
- post-traumatic stress disorder
- depression
- obsessive-compulsive disorder
- pain relief
- end-stage psychotherapy with the dying (mostly cancer and more recently AIDS)
- facilitation of the meditative state
- elicitation of mystical experience

There are currently five schedules (or categories) into which drugs are placed in U.S. legislative practice (see page 133). It is not the scheduling criteria that are problematic; rather, it is the politics of how and why drugs are placed in a particular schedule that is flawed. So psychedelics and marijuana are placed in Schedule 1, although neither is as addictive (if at all) as heroin, with which they are categorized, and both have medicinal value. They have been placed in Schedule 1 for fear-based political reasons, not on an objective scientific, medical basis.

FIVE U.S. DRUG SCHEDULES AND PLACEMENT CRITERIA

Schedule I, including LSD, heroin, cannabis

▶ The drug or other substance has a high potential for abuse.

▶ The drug or other substance has no currently accepted medical use in treatment in the United States.

▶ There is a lack of accepted safety for use of the drug or other substance under medical supervision.

Schedule II, including cocaine, meperidine, Tuinal, methadone

▶ The drug or other substance has a high potential for abuse.

▶ The drug or other substance has a currently accepted medical use in treatment in the United States or a currently accepted medical use with severe restrictions.

▶ Abuse of the drug or other substances may lead to severe psychological or physical dependence.

Schedule III, including amphetamine, phencyclidine, Pentothal, lysergic acid

▶ The drug or other substance has a potential for abuse less than the drugs or other substances in Schedules I and II.

▶ The drug or other substance has a currently accepted medical use in treatment in the United States.

▶ Abuse of the drug or other substance may lead to moderate or low physical dependence or high psychological dependence.

Schedule IV, including phenobarbital, meprobamate

▶ The drug or other substance has a low potential for abuse relative to the drugs or other substances in Schedule III.

▶ The drug or other substance has a currently accepted medical use in treatment in the United States.

▶ Abuse of the drug or other substance may lead to limited physical dependence or psychological dependence relative to the drugs or other substances in Schedule III.

Schedule V, including dilutions and admixtures of scheduled drugs or substances

▶ The drug or other substance has a low potential for abuse relative to the drugs or other substances in Schedule IV.

▶ The drug or other substance has a currently accepted medical use in treatment in the United States.

▶ Abuse of the drug or other substance may lead to limited physical dependence or psychological dependence relative to the drugs or other substances in Schedule IV.

While the "Five U.S. Drug Schedules and Placement Criteria" lists three selection criteria—abuse potential, currently accepted medical use, and safety/dependence potential—there are actually eight more detailed factors that are supposed to be used in determining Schedule placement:

1. Drug or substance actual or relative potential for abuse
2. Scientific evidence of its pharmacological effect, if known
3. The state of current scientific knowledge regarding the drug or other substance
4. Its history and current pattern of abuse
5. The scope, duration, and significance of abuse
6. What, if any, risk there is to the public health
7. Its psychic or physiological dependence liability
8. Whether the substance is an immediate precursor of a substance already controlled

Of the eight factors, the only consideration that could be construed as negative in the placement of psychedelics are those that contain the word *abuse*. Yet *abuse* is a subjective term and can be a self-fulfilling prophecy: if psychedelics are not considered therapeutic (and are in a Schedule where it has until recently been very difficult to conduct human-subjects clinical research to demonstrate therapeutic efficacy), then provision of psychedelic therapy will be defined perforce to be abuse. Even further, if use of psychedelics by the public is categorized as illegal, then personal spiritual exploration will likewise be considered to be abuse. Beyond these factors, in making scheduling decisions we must also consider certain ethical issues, such as: the right of the dying to determine their own treatment, especially after all other treatments have failed and had to be abandoned; the right of all humans to cognitive liberty and, further, to cognitive enhancement (when not a danger to self or others—but again, that subjective term, *abuse* comes into play in defining *danger*); and the right, enshrined in the U.S. Constitution

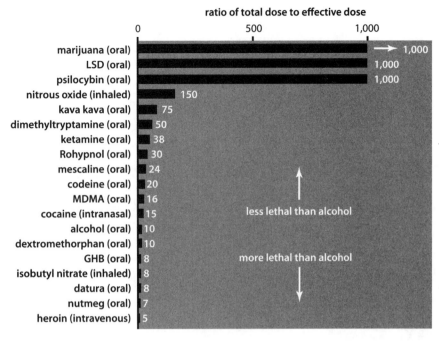

Figure 5.1. This table shows the fatality-to-effectiveness ratio for various drugs, which is a measure of safety. The psychedelics tend to have the greatest safety margins, and the depressant drugs, such as heroin, the lowest margins of safety. Is there any reason, any logical justification, to place psychedelics in the same schedule as heroin?

(and more recently reestablished and strengthened in the Religious Freedom Restoration Act) to unfettered freedom to determine our own religious practices.

The table shown in figure 5.2 on page 134 gives a more detailed picture, but arrives at the same conclusion. From the perspective of physical harm, dependence potential, or even broad measures of "social harm," psychedelics are relatively safe, compared with other, often less stringently scheduled drugs of potential misuse.[13]

So if we are to reschedule psychedelics, which one or ones will be rescheduled first and to which schedule will they be reassigned? The table below provides a comparison of the pros and cons of the currently researched psychedelics.

	Physical harm				Dependence				Social Harm			
	Mean	Acute	Chronic	Intravenous	Mean	Pleasure	Psychological dependence	Physical dependence	Mean	Intoxication	Social harm	Health-care costs
Heroin	2.78	2.8	2.5	3.0	3.00	3.0	3.0	3.0	2.54	1.6	3.0	3.0
Cocaine	2.33	2.0	2.0	3.0	2.39	3.0	2.8	1.3	2.17	1.8	2.5	2.3
Barbituates	2.23	2.3	1.9	2.5	2.01	2.0	2.2	1.8	2.00	2.4	1.9	1.7
Street methadone	1.86	2.5	1.7	1.4	2.08	1.8	3.2	2.3	1.87	1.6	1.9	2.0
Alcohol	1.40	1.9	2.4	NA	2.3	1.9	1.6	2.21	2.2	2.4	2.1	2.1
Ketamine	2.00	2.1	1.7	2.1	1.54	1.9	1.7	1.0	1.69	2.0	1.5	1.5
Benzodiazepines	1.63	1.5	1.7	1.8	1.83	1.7	2.1	1.8	1.65	2.0	1.5	1.5
Amphetamine	1.81	1.3	1.8	2.4	1.67	2.0	1.9	1.1	1.50	1.4	1.5	1.6
Tobacco	1.24	0.9	2.9	0	2.21	2.3	2.6	1.8	1.42	0.8	1.1	2.4
Buprenorphine	1.6	1.2	1.3	2.3	1.64	2.0	1.5	1.5	1.49	1.6	1.5	1.4
Cannabis	0.99	0.9	2.1	0	1.51	1.9	1.7	0.8	1.50	1.7	1.3	1.5
Solvents	1.28	2.1	1.7	0.	1.01	1.7	1.2	0.1	1.52	1.9	1.5	1.2
4-MTA	1.44	2.2	2.1	0.	1.30	1.0	1.7	0.8	1.06	1.2	1.0	1.0
LSD	1.13	1.7	1.4	0.3	1.23	2.2	1.1	0.3	1.32	1.6	1.3	1.1
Methylphenidate	1.32	1.2	1.3	1.6	1.25	1.4	1.3	1.0	0.97	1.1	0.8	1.1
Anabolic steriods	1.45	0.8	2.0	1.7	0.88	1.1	0.8	0.8	1.13	1.3	0.8	1.3
GHB	0.86	1.4	1.2	0	1.19	1.4	1.1	1.1	1.30	1.4	1.3	1.2
Ecstasy	1.05	1.6	1.6	0	1.13	1.5	1.2	0.7	1.09	1.2	1.0	1.1
Alkylnitrites	0.93	1.6	0.9	0.3	0.87	1.6	0.7	0.3	0.97	0.8	0.7	1.4
Khat	0.50	0.3	1.2	0	1.04	1.6	1.2	0.3	0.85	0.7	1.1	0.8

Figure 5.2. Table showing the mean independent group scores in each of the three categories of harm, for 20 substances, ranked by their overall score, and mean scores for each of the three subscales. From Nutt et al., 2007.

PROS AND CONS OF RESCHEDULING VARIOUS PSYCHEDELICS

	PROS	CONS
Psilocybin	established physiological safety; powerful, but relatively manageable; useful for end-of-life anxiety	can be moderately psychologically challenging
MDMA	anxiolytic; good PTSD application	physiologically demanding; high toxicity-to-effectiveness ratio
LSD	powerful/effective; physiologically nontoxic (no known lethal dose)	intensity; long course of action (can be a plus); notoriety/fear
DMT	very short acting (too short?); Strassman's ground work; connection to ayahuasca	intensity; otherworldly, difficult to integrate; connection to ayahuasca
DPT	relatively short acting; Spring Grove ground work	under researched (can be a plus); Spring Grove saw as less effective than LSD
Ketamine	already Schedule III, short acting	dissociative, difficult to integrate

As of this writing, it seems like it is becoming a beautiful horse race between psilocybin and MDMA, as they are both being used in research and producing excellent results. A related question then emerges: to which schedule they should be moved? Schedule I contains the only set of drugs that may not be prescribed by a physician, meaning that even a move to Schedule II (a tightly controlled category containing cocaine, Demerol, and methadone) would enable the prescription use of psychedelics. In addition, rescheduling psychedelics to Schedule II or III would enable prescription for off-label use, that is, for medical purposes other than those for which the drug was originally approved. This would mean that if MDMA became a Schedule II drug approved for use with post-traumatic stress disorder, it could also be used for, say, relationship therapy (conducted by a psychiatrist). Again, with positive research results and lots of young psychiatrists newly trained in the therapeutic use of psychedelics, this type of rescheduling is necessary, likely, and will open up a new age of psychedelic therapy. One important caveat is that we must be scrupulously cautious about not allowing these most powerful of psychiatric drugs to be misused, either by psychiatrists or by escaping the professional context as they did in the 1960s. Such a development could prove disastrous for this fledgling field.

WHY DO PSYCHEDELICS PROVIDE PAIN RELIEF FOR THE DYING?

Between 1963 and 1967, psychiatrist Eric Kast published several papers documenting his pioneering work administering LSD to the dying at the Chicago Medical School. For fifty cancer patients with gangrene, Kast compared Dilaudid, Demerol, and LSD for pain relief. The Dilaudid provided three hours of pain relief, the Demerol lasted for two hours, and remarkably the LSD lasted an astonishing ninety-two hours and up to ten days in certain instances.[14] With LSD, the analgesic effect came on slower, but lasted significantly longer. In Kast's next study, with 128 patients, the pain disappeared for twelve hours with LSD and was reduced for two to three weeks.[15] In Kast's last study, eighty patients were treated with LSD. Seventy-two percent said it was at least "pleasant"; 85 percent said they'd take it again; and 72 percent said they had had important insights. Kast explained these results as "the attenuation of anticipation" in his patient subjects. He theorized that the anticipation of their death provoked anxiety in his patients, which was met with denial via sublimation, and abreaction transposed their anticipatory anxiety into physical symptoms, predominantly pain. According to Kast, the overwhelming nature of the psychedelic experience distracted patients from their anticipation of death, thus reducing felt anxiety and so the need for its transposition into pain.[16] (Further research will be required to determine whether an unknown pain modulation mechanism of the serotonergic system could be responsible for the pain relief observed.)

Beginning in 1965, Pahnke, Grof, Yensen, and others at the Research Unit of the Spring Grove State Hospital (and after 1969, in the Clinical Sciences Department of the Maryland Psychiatric Research Center) conducted psychedelic research with cancer patients. These researchers found the analgesia not so much associated with dose, but with peak experience. They also found that even among the group that had a peak experience, the analgesic effect was not reliably replicable. What was replicable, however, was a change in attitude toward death among those with a peak experience. With a change in attitude and a freer airing and acceptance of certain family issues, the relationship with the family was often also improved, resulting in a more peaceful death.[17]

Another example of research on the healing effect of the peak experience in psychedelic therapy may be found in the last works of Walter Pahnke. Working with the most advanced researchers at the most advanced psychedelic research facility of its day (the Maryland Psychiatric Research Center), Pahnke (a minister and a physician with Harvard degrees) gave LSD to seventeen dying patients. The subjects were given intensive therapeutic preparation, with lots of TLC. Two-thirds had dramatic or moderate improvement in tension, depression, pain, and fear of death—but there was no control group. Their conclusion was that both drug and suggestion were required for a peak experience.[18] Kast, on the other hand, didn't give any preparation or TLC (beyond standard bedside manner) and still got excellent results. The explanation, of course, is not an issue of either/or, but rather a matter of degree. Either drug alone, or suggestion alone, may lead to a peak experience, but giving both simultaneously will more reliably do so.[19]

Stanislav Grof wrote an influential book with anthropologist Joan Halifax called *The Human Encounter with Death,* based on his work at the Spring Grove and Maryland Psychiatric facilities. Grof and Halifax describe the analgesic effect of psychedelics as unpredictable, but the philosophical, psychospiritual effects as more profound and long lasting.

They hypothesized, similar to Kast, that the reason these people had such an extraordinary analgesic effect from LSD was not because LSD is an analgesic, per se. In this culture, it is much more acceptable to say, "I hurt physically—give me a drug to relieve the pain," than it is to say, "I'm terrified of dying, and there's nothing you can do for me." As such, it was hypothesized that a proportion of the pain involved in a cancer death is actually displaced fear of dying. When patients have a peak LSD experience (or potentially any experience that reduces fear of death, such as a transformative spiritual event or near-death experience), they have less need to displace their anxiety into more socially acceptable pain symptoms and so the felt degree of physical pain can decrease.

Psychedelic research with the dying was the last to stop and has justifiably become among the first to start again (with research on easing end-of-life anxiety in cancer patients under way at Harvard using MDMA and at UCLA, Johns Hopkins, and NYU using psilocybin). The issue of short-term effect, with the attendant need for booster shots, is less of an issue with the dying—a short-term effect is all that is sought. Yet there is a danger of developing a subtly cavalier attitude in dealing with the dying. A negative result has no less negative impact just because the subjects will be dead shortly after treatment. In fact, a negative result is worse for a subject with precious little time to sort out a sad or confusing experience. Even so, the potential to reduce the fear and even the physical pain experienced by the dying, to improve family relations so fewer die angry or estranged, to provide a peaceful state of mind in the weeks before death—these are the kinds of suggestive early findings that cry out for careful further research.[20]

CAN PSYCHEDELICS PROVIDE LASTING CHANGE?

Use new drugs quickly, while they still work.

ARMAND TROUSSEAU, NINETEENTH-CENTURY

FRENCH INTERNIST

Clinical research has demonstrated the effective use of psychedelics in all of the categories of application listed above. Yet, to generalize, the data do not show permanent effects.

In criminal recidivism, for example, Timothy Leary, while still an instructor at Harvard, did a fascinating study at the Concord Correctional Facility in Massachusetts, showing a 25 percent recidivism rate for the first six months after treatment, versus 64 percent for the general prison population. (Even these findings have been called into question by Doblin's 1998 review of Leary's original data, which found some fudging of the numbers.) Twenty-four months later, however, no difference in recidivism was seen.[21]

In Arendsen Hein's pioneering work with LSD in Holland, two-thirds of his most difficult cases were improved in his 1963 study.[22] In his 1972 follow-up, he was so disappointed that he recommended that psychedelics be used primarily with the dying—because you don't have to worry as much about the effect fading.[23]

In the research literature on alcoholism, we repeatedly see moderate to dramatic improvement in hard-core alcoholics six months after treatment with psychedelics, but in later follow-up, the rates of alcoholism are similar to those before treatment.[24] Clearly, we are seeing short-term gains that are not sustained. The one-shot, silver bullet, miracle cure, psychedelic therapy dream was wishful thinking and just hasn't panned out. This type of treatment effect can be profound and potentially life changing, but proves to be short term. However, we don't expect penicillin to work in one dose and we don't expect insulin to be a short-term treatment resulting in a cure. We accept that penicillin must be taken repeatedly over a period of time and that insulin is required on an ongoing basis. The answer may be to give booster shots over time. If subjects are abstinent at six months post-treatment, but back off the wagon at two years, that's a wonderful finding! What other treatment can claim the six-month effect? If this treatment is to be adopted, implemented, and sustained over the long term, this finding indicates the need for a public policy of taking the medication on an ongoing, periodic basis.

The Native American Church (NAC) provides a good example of an ongoing "treatment." Although there is a high frequency of alcoholism among Native Americans, members of the NAC take peyote on a regular basis and have a very low alcoholism rate. No drinking is permitted among church members, and they view the peyote ceremony as being part of the cure for alcoholism.[25] Of course, these are only suggestive, correlational findings, and yet the NAC and the South American–based ayahuasca churches, UDV and Santo Daime, all represent "natural experiments," the results of which must be carefully considered in creating policies in the U.S. for psychedelic therapy and sacramental use.[26]

CAN PSYCHEDELICS INDUCE REAL SPIRITUALITY?

Scholars of the origins of religion have speculated that hunter-gatherers foraging for roots and berries would surely have ingested psychedelic plants and shortly thereafter experienced what may have been our first intimations of spiritual consciousness.[27] There is no proof of that, but it is an intriguing theory.

In contemporary research, subjects do, in fact, report mystical and peak experiences.[28] Masters and Houston's classic research on 202 subjects found 96 percent experienced religious imagery; 3 percent reported a full mystical experience; 40 percent had less fear of death; 60 percent had increased trust in God—or in life, if they were atheists.[29] This finding was correlated with the dose, set, and the setting: religious music and iconography increased the likelihood of a peak experience.[30]

Masters and Houston treated 206 subjects with LSD or mescaline and identified four levels of a psychedelic experience. The mildest, or earliest, level is *sensory-perceptual*—wherein visual distortions and other sensory phenomena predominate. The second level, stronger, deeper, and later in onset, is what Masters and Houston called *recollective-analytic*—covering childhood memories and psychological issues. The third level is the *symbolic*—with a focus on archetypes, the ecological, the mythic, and the global. The fourth and final level is what they called *integrative*—a full-blown mystical experience.

Yet these stages of intensity of psychedelic experience don't vary based only on increasing dose, as one might expect. In addition, a peak or "religious" experience is more likely to occur as time progresses over the course of a single trip (e.g., in psychedelic therapy), as familiarity with psychedelics increases over time (e.g., in the course of psycholytic psychotherapy), and as experience and maturity increase over years of use. Emphasis tends to be on the sensory and perceptual first, moving on over time, dose, experience, and so forth, toward the ecstatic. This progression parallels the stages of developmental psychology, with the successive loss of egocentrism, as well as the developmental sequence laid out in yogic chakra levels, which move from personal bodily and other material concerns, through compassion for others, to spiritual unity with the universe. As such, the early, sensory-perceptual stage of "pretty colors" may be seen as a curtain of beads occupying the immature until such time as they are developmentally ready to move on to other levels of psychedelic experience and spiritual development.

Walter Pahnke, for his doctorate in religion and society at Harvard University, conducted the third Leary study we will describe. Referred to as "The Miracle at Marsh Chapel" or "The Good Friday Experiment," Pahnke's study used twenty divinity students, together as a group in a strongly religious setting (the basement of Boston University's Marsh Chapel, with a Good Friday sermon being piped in from the chapel above). Half the subjects received 30 milligrams of psilocybin (a large dose) and half got an active placebo comprising nicotinic acid, which gives a flushing sensation, and Benzedrine, in a double-blind design. Forty-five minutes into the experiment, it became obvious who had received the placebo and who had received the experimental treatment.

In analyzing the results, Pahnke used the work of W. T. Stace, a philosopher of religion, who had identified seven characteristics of the mystical experience: unitary consciousness; nonspatial, nontemporal awareness; sense of reality and objectivity to the experience; blessedness; sacredness; paradoxicality; and ineffability—the inability to describe it. Pahnke added two more, transiency and subsequent life improvement, for a total of nine characteristics of the mystical experience to use as a measure in the study.[31]

The results showed five of the ten who received the active treatment were significant in all nine of the categories. Nine of the ten reported having a true religious experience. Although the double-blind was blown as soon as the psychedelic took effect, the use of a control group still helped by equalizing expectations—and thus the crucial variable of anticipatory mind-set—between the control and experimental groups early on, before the drug took effect.

There was a long-term follow-up done in 1987 on the study subjects.[32] Seven out of the ten who had the active dose and nine control subjects were found. Of the experimental subjects, all said they had a positive time and all preferred nondrug routes to mysticism. One of the experimental subjects actually had a bad trip in the experiment, seeing Christ on the cross, and getting into a fervor that was pathological to the point where the experimenters had to give him Thorazine to come down. That was not reported in the original research by Leary.

This again brings up the point that these are serious, powerful substances—and that users become very susceptible to suggestion. With research conducted in a church, it makes sense that someone would start to believe they see—or are—Christ.

In a recent, meticulously designed study, Roland Griffiths and colleagues at Johns Hopkins University replicated Pahnke's results, with twenty-four of thirty-six volunteers reporting a "complete mystical" experience with psilocybin, compared with four of thirty-five controls receiving an active placebo.[33]

Even in studies that scrupulously avoid religious imagery and iconography, subjects still report spiritual experiences. In Oscar Janiger's pioneering research with LSD in a neutral, nonreligious environment, 24 percent of the volunteers reported experiences that "resonate closely with classic descriptions of spiritual transcendence."[34]

Yet the psychedelic experience is triggered by the ingestion of a substance and, since that means of provoking a religious experience is not accepted today, many question whether the mystical experience achieved while on a psychedelic is a *real* religious experience. From our postmodern perspective, it is difficult to separate conscious experience from neurochemistry. Is what is going on in my brain right now my will, or is it my chemistry? Not just psychedelics, but fasting, breathing exercises, prolonged wakefulness, isolation, self-flagellation, martial arts, prayer, and meditation—all these things can bring about a profound mystical experience. Many of these techniques were used by the prophets of the Hebrew Scriptures—were they "real" religious experiences, if they were purposely triggered or provoked?

Aldous Huxley called the experience of psychedelics "a gratuitous grace."[35] Huxley saw psychedelic epiphany as a gift—not earned, not necessary or sufficient for salvation—to be enjoyed as a window into enlightenment. He called his book *The Doors of Perception* (after William Blake's line in *The Marriage of Heaven and Hell*: "But first the notion that man has a body distinct from his soul is to be expunged. . . . If the doors of perception were cleansed every thing would appear to man as it is, infinite").

Even so, psychedelics are more a window than a door; they provide the opportunity to experience the profound beauty and wholeness reported by the mystic, but only for a brief period of chemically provoked vision. On psychedelics we may see heaven, but we may not take up residence there. As an analogy, consider being on a path up a mountain. We are high up and the clouds are so thick that we can't really see more than a yard or two in front of us. We can continue on our path, but we certainly cannot see the peak of the mountain, which is always obscured by clouds. After a while, we begin to question whether the goal is really there at all and whether it is still worth going forward. Psychedelics, under the right conditions, can offer a temporary parting of the clouds, the ability to see the peak with great clarity for a brief period of time. After the experience is gone and the clouds come back, we can't see that peak anymore, but we still vividly remember that it does in fact exist. That part of the experience is lasting.

Although sustainability of the visionary state is a limiting problem, there is no method as predictable in producing a spiritual experience, or as potent in impact, as psychedelic chemicals. Of all the other methods mentioned—fasting, flagellation, meditation, and the rest—none are as effective and reliable as psychedelics in producing a visionary state. That is why they've been used for that purpose by every civilization known to have had access to them, with the sad exception of Western civilization (and the Inuit, who have no psychoactive plants or animals in their arctic environment). In practical terms, psychedelics are and always have been ubiquitous—they become a problem when people trip repeatedly to try to sustain that mystical experience, because it doesn't last. A drug-induced religious experience is not the same thing as making the effort, over time, to develop a spiritual life.

A psychedelic trip, especially when one has had a dissociative, ego-death experience, is one of life's most extreme states of mind, but so is a high fever or a near-death experience in an automobile accident, when people may see their life flash before their eyes. These drugs have been called "nonspecific catalysts and amplifiers of the psyche."[36] Their effect is largely determined by the context in which they're given and the expectations of the user and the giver. How much of the therapeutic effect of psychedelics is a result of the chemical, the intensity of the experience, or the psychology of the patient? We need follow-up research to address these important and frustratingly unanswered questions.

To summarize, then, in terms of spirituality, it is quite clear that subjects do, indeed, report spiritual experiences: 24 to 96 percent in several studies, depending on the set and setting. The question that frequently arises next is: Is the peak experience derived from psychedelic drugs a real spiritual experience or a type of chemical mimicry? There has been much debate on that issue, and I'll not try to resolve it here.[37] In general, however, people who have experienced psychedelics are more likely to be among the camp who claim that it is a real spiritual experience, and those who claim it is not a real experience tend to be those who have not experienced psychedelics personally.

How do we separate mystical experience from the underlying neurochemical substrate? All our bodily and psychological phenomenology is mediated by what happens in the brain. In reality, we don't experience the outside world: rather, our experience is of internal neurochemicals released by the brain in response to electrical signals triggered by incoming stimuli from the outside world.[38]

Many people have noticed that there is a consistent worldview that visionaries, seers, and gurus see and report back: unitive, transcendent, accepting, transphysical, indescribable, infinite, joyful, whole.[39] Moreover, the visionaries, seers, and gurus have pointed consistently to the many ways to get there: meditation, drugs, fasting, mortification of the flesh and self-flagellation, rituals, trance, rhythmic drumming, focusing incantations, mantras, spells, breathing exercises, prolonged wakefulness, sensory deprivation, carbon dioxide buildup in the blood, martial arts, prayer, and so on. All these techniques have been used to induce a profound mystical experience, with marked accompanying changes in brain chemistry. So, is what's going on in your brain right now *will*, or is it chemistry? Or are those simply two perspectives of the same thing—two different levels on our conceptual resolving microscope?

If we are indeed moving to an integral worldview in which chemistry and spirituality are seen as mirrored perspectives of our essential wholeness, then we are also moving toward a world where medicines are used not only to heal sickness, but also to facilitate personal growth among the healthy.[40] As has been the case for the past fifty years, the Baby Boom generation of entitled seekers will help spur this transformation in government policy, from sickness medicines to the even bigger market for wellness medicines. Clearly, the pharmaceutical companies would be eager for a huge new market, and so scientists and regulators must consider hard the consequences of permitting the manipulation of our own genetic biochemical endowment. This is especially the case as advanced technologies such as Positron Emission Tomography (PET), functional Magnetic Resonance Imaging (fMRI), wide-field fluorescence microscopy, laser scanning confocal microscopy (LSCM), live-cell confocal and high-resolution deconvolution microscopy, and intelligent computer modeling eventually will enable us to specify all actual and potential relationships between the structure of our neural receptor sites and the activity that would result from all possible chemical fits. Once we have specified the nature of all structure-activity relationships (SARs), we will be immeasurably more vulnerable to unscrupulous governmental or commercial organizations bent on control and exploitation.[41] If psychedelic peak experience psychotherapy does induce a true spiritual experience, as subjects claim, then are psychedelics most appropriately in the purview of physicians and scientists or of the clergy? The San Francisco-based Council on Spiritual Practices is interested in what they call *entheogens*—substances that engender the spiritual within us. Founder Robert Jesse is working with theologians because he feels that these substances are sacraments that should be reintroduced into established religions and used without medical administration (after medical screening).[42]

Psychedelic research has gained enormous sophistication over the years in grappling with methodological and theoretical issues such as these. If psychedelics can be demonstrated, more or less reliably, to induce spiritual experience, how might that capability be helpful in medicine and to society? The answer lies in the mystical experience—or, for the atheist—Maslow's "peak experience" variable. The gut intention is always the source of healing and the agent of change. Miracles literally do happen only to those who believe. Whether it's alcoholism, marital discord, end-of-life anxiety, or even meditation, with psychedelics triggering the core to release, it becomes, for the alcoholic: "Oh, my God, I've wasted my life on alcohol, but it's not too late"; for the marriage in trouble: "Oh, my God, now I remember why I fell in love with her all those years ago!"; for the late-stage cancer patient: "Oh, my

God, I'm dying and I'm estranged from my only brother! But it's not too late to make amends"; or for the meditator, simply: "Oh, my God!" The commonality, of course, is the dramatic, life-review type of experience in which one's mortality is primary and connection to the entire universe, often with a superior being, is central. Those people are more likely to be "cured."

So it seems it is fundamentally the numinous, the ineffable—the spiritual—that has the ability to take our entire life force, our total self and bodily energy, and focus it on a deeply felt need, such as healing. In other words, the profound spiritual feelings engendered by psychedelics are nothing less than the *über* vehicle for healing, the underlying driving force behind the body's natural healing process, operative in spontaneous remission or a miraculous cure. If healing is fundamentally mind over matter, it must always—can only—emanate from the whole grounded power of our core, the psyche, the "gut." If we are careful moving forward, psychedelics may be able to offer society a safe and effective means to access what we think of as the psyche, the soul, or the core of our being, and as we align ourselves with that foundation, they may enable us to heal inside, as well as in our relationships and our society as a whole.

What would such a worldview be like and how might we attain it? That is the topic for the next chapter.

6

THE DEVELOPMENT OF AN INTEGRAL CLINICAL APPROACH

I have found that there are two approaches to peace of mind. One is transcendent, the other, cathartic.

TRANSCENDENCE VS. THE FRONTAL ASSAULT

The transcendent model holds that approaching one's formative past directly, say, through discussion about one's childhood experience with parents, tends to engender resistance. I call this the "frontal assault" approach, and it doesn't work. I compare it to chasing a ferret.

Ferrets are remarkable creatures. Fast and wily, they are notoriously difficult to capture and tame. Imagine that we are chasing a ferret across the prairie, and it runs under a rock outcropping. We finally have it cornered! We reach under the outcropping and the ferret backs in farther. We reach in even more, and the ferret retreats all the way to the back of the little cave. We reach in farther, and WRAWR! the ferret lashes out, cutting our hand. This is what happens when we try to retrieve a painful memory directly.

Here is another approach. We see the ferret run under the rock outcropping. We sit down six feet or so away from the cave. We open our backpack and take out our lunch. We cut off a small chunk of meat and throw it at the opening of the little cave and we wait. Nothing is expected at first, but eventually the ferret sneaks up, quickly grabs the piece of meat, and scoots back to the safety in the back. We sit and throw another piece of meat toward the cave opening. We wait. Of course, the outcome of this little parable is that eventually, a week, a month, a year later, the ferret is sitting in your lap, being hand-fed slices of meat.

So it is with our painful, protected memories and associations (or analyses): if we set up a safe and rewarding environment, over time repressed issues will come to light in a relaxed way.

This is the opposite of the "frontal assault" approach—this is the "bottom-up" approach: don't even try to get inside the subconscious in a top-down process. There's too much resistance. Rather, come in below the personality, below the defensive persona, right down at the level of the core issue of fear and love, and provide safe, trusted love.

This is the equivalent of the way I would take psychedelics. In chapter 1, I described my first trip of what I think of as "the modern era"—my adult, postcollege rediscovery of psychedelics for personal development. I describe how at the beginning of this first trip in almost twenty years, I tried to examine my "roots" and they recoiled away from my scrutiny, but that I came to an attitude of compassion and acceptance when I touched the glowing orb at the ground of my being. Then, when I gazed again upon my roots, but with empathy, they relaxed and opened up to my total acceptance.

There was only one problem with that approach: it didn't last.

While the experience of viewing my deepest childhood issues with loving compassion, the experience of being seen with such loving compassion, is a deeply relaxing experience that enables the true, sweet, original, childhood self to emerge from hiding—to come out from under the rock outcropping, up from the basement, out from under the boulder—that feeling tends to fade in the days following the trip. The defensive structure of the strategic personality reemerges, like "memory metal." Memory metal is an alloy that "remembers" its original, cold, forged shape and that returns to that shape after being deformed by applying heat. Sounds a lot like what happens in "the heat" of a trip and then after, as the experience cools.

Alan Watts famously said of tripping repeatedly: "When you get the message, hang up the phone," meaning that repeated tripping isn't the path to enlightenment. Yet, no one asks insulin to be a silver bullet; perhaps the effects of psychedelics are best maintained through "booster shots"—periodic readministration, coupled with psychodynamic psychotherapy and/or meditation. At least this was my emerging thinking until I found catharsis at Burning Man in 2007.

CATHARSIS, OR HOW I COMPLETED MY CHILDHOOD AT BURNING MAN

My first visit to Burning Man was at the request of Rick Doblin, founder and executive director of the Multidisciplinary Association for Psychedelic Studies (MAPS). Rick had invited me out to serve as a counselor or sitter at Sanctuary in the past, but I had always demurred, thinking that the conditions (arid, 100°F temperatures, dust storms, minimal services) would be too uncomfortable and that the twenty-four-hour party atmosphere was not my preference. After a few years of requests, I felt an obligation to support Rick, so I agreed to work at Sanctuary. The night before my trip to Burning Man, I was up very late packing all my gear and, nervous as to what I'd encounter, slept very little. On arrival, I found that we were camped next to a huge, all-night dance installation with driving, ear-splitting, diaphragm-throbbing bass music starting at 4 p.m. and continuing without stop until 10 a.m. Although I did have earplugs, and they worked, they did nothing to stop the throb, throb, throbbing of the music through my body all night. I felt like a snare drum vibrating without being struck. Of course, I didn't sleep that night either. I woke up despairing of my ability to last a week under those circumstances. How could I go on without any sleep? Could I give up and slink away with my tail between my legs, when so many people were successfully navigating the demands of the desert—and seemed to be having a great time doing it?

That morning was the orientation meeting for Sanctuary workers. As I walked to the session through the dust,* I wondered how and why I had gotten myself into this mess. The shower in the RV was broken, the toilet was already unusable, and the showers at my campground— Entheon Village, run by MAPS and CoSM (artist Alex Grey's Chapel of Sacred Mirrors)—weren't set up yet. I was alone, sleep deprived, and dirty.

As if arriving at an oasis, at the Sanctuary orientation I found a collection of the most loving, warm, helpful, compassionate people I'd ever met. This was a tent full of angels—people with smiles on their faces, sitting, munching, drinking water, smoking cannabis, all the while welcoming me, inquiring about my story, sharing their own—preparing for the heart-filling opportunity to help others. I felt as if for the first time in my adult life, I was with people who felt, thought, and acted like me, who shared the same values and sweet tendencies to help and learn; I felt as if I'd met my people, as if I'd found home. I had attended a training session in New York in the weeks prior to arrival at Burning Man, but this orientation was necessary too and extremely helpful. I was told, "Sanctuary work isn't about doing psychedelic therapy. It's about creating a safe container—a nest—for people having a difficult psychedelic experience, or just a difficult Burning Man experience." In Sanctuary, we provide a space where it is safe for anyone to play out their process—as long as they aren't a danger to themselves or others—in a way that, were they to do it out on the Playa, could get them sedated (bad enough), or sedated, restrained, and taken away from Burning Man in an (expensive) ambulance.

---

*The dust storms at Burning Man are legendary. Dust pervades everything, with or without a storm. In one's shoes, under one's nails, regardless of how frequently one might want to clean or sweep, the dust covers every surface of every tent, RV, or service area, and as you might expect, finds its way into every human orifice, every crack, everywhere. Face masks and hand creams are essential . . . and essentially useless against the onslaught.

As I left that meeting, I had one of the most unusual experiences of my life. Feeling elated by my sense of finding a community of angels to nest among, yet being stung by the dry, hot dust of yet another gritty windstorm, I walked back to my campground with tears streaming out of my eyes and a broad, ear-to-ear smile covering my face—laughing and crying at the same time! That phenomenology nicely sums up the Burning Man experience: one is broken down and raised up. This breaking down of my power to control events in my life, coupled with the dharmic beauty of the people around me, helped prepare me for the facilitated psychedelic experience I had the day of the Burn, one of only a few permanently transformative psychedelic experiences I've ever had.

Burning Man is a "time out of time": despite the federal, state, local, and Bureau of Land Management officers making their presence known (the festival is held on federal land), they generally do not intrude on the activities.* In this freewheeling context, it is predictable that in addition to Sanctuary workers who help those having a difficult experience with psychedelics at Burning Man, there are also those who choose to help others who intentionally decide they want guidance for a planned psychedelic session. Being a one-shot experience, this is not psychedelic therapy, but a planned growth experience. The assistance is more than simply sitting with the tripper—it's meant to be an active, often difficult, and hopefully rewarding, perhaps even transformative, experience. So it was no surprise to me when I was approached by a colleague and asked if I would be interested in acting as such a guide. After only a

---

*For example, if an officer smells marijuana coming from a tent off the main path, they will generally not intervene. If an attendee walks up to an officer and asks for a light, the officer will issue what they themselves refer to as a "Stupid Tax"—a fine for being in possession of a controlled substance. The same is true of dangerous behavior on the Playa. Unless a felony is being committed, the law enforcement authorities will generally look for "Rangers"—Burning Man's own trained and universally accepted "hall monitors"—to intercede. Rangers are trained to take a laissez faire approach to just about everything short of potentially fatal behavior—and even that is not actively prevented, if it is only the actor who will die and others' lives are not threatened by the dangerous behavior. The theme of Burning Man is always "radical self-reliance"—food, water, and shelter are not provided—and that theme generally applies to policing attendees' behavior as well.

moment's thought, I responded that while I would like to be helpful, I felt unqualified to be a guide in this capacity.* On the other hand, I was eager to be on the receiving end of this offer, that is, to have a guided experience in the safety of others who regularly, selflessly did this sort of thing. It was arranged that on the day of the Burn, Saturday, I would have a psychedelic session with a former underground therapist I had known and trusted for fifteen years and a Canadian clinical psychiatrist who studied these substances, whom I met and trusted immediately.

As the day approached, I wondered what would emerge from the experience. I continued my "safe container" work at the Sanctuary and also acted as emcee for the psychedelic speakers program at Entheon Village that I curated with Rick Doblin and gave a presentation there, but when I wasn't working, my mind was focused on the facilitated experience, speculating on just what I had signed up for and what I might see.

On the day of the session, I came to the appointed location: a round, tall tent, some twenty-five feet across, with overlapping carpets spread everywhere. I settled in with my notebook, blanket, and water. I took a somewhat larger amount of mushrooms than usual and began to chat with my therapist-guides about what we wanted to focus on and what our expectations were. I began to tell them about how I tripped, about the roots of my psychology recoiling from my picking and analysis, and about bypassing my psychological issues at the beginning of a trip, until I'd touched that throbbing orb at the ground of my being, when everything would be accepted and my problems would be transformed into poignant developmental challenges. I concluded that I would need some time at the beginning to get to that place, and so I was going to go inside now and would come back up to work with them on those

---

*Due to the laws against it, I have never been trained to conduct a psychedelic session. No one has since the 1960s, as there are currently no training programs, other than in research projects, for psychedelic therapists (and those trained in the early days are not permitted to work as therapists in private practice). So, as I tell the many people who contact me for such services, I cannot ethically provide psychedelic therapy.

challenges in about an hour. They looked at each other with bemused astonishment and said, "Go there now." I replied that they didn't understand and explained again about the roots, the glowing orb, the ground of my being . . . and they responded, "Go there now." I began to get frustrated and irritated—disillusioned by their inability to understand the beauty, and effectiveness, of what I was trying to do. They asked how I was feeling, and I told them that I was disappointed at having to teach them—the experts—such a simple thing. I could see that they were becoming frustrated with me, with my arrogance and my resistance; they even told me I was beginning to waste their time.

At this point I knew that I was making my psychedelic psychotherapists mad at me—not a good idea when you're coming on to a psychedelic state (and at this point, I was feeling the mushrooms quite strongly). So I gave in and said, "OK. What do you want me to do?" They said, "Go there now." Frustrated still but resigned to place myself in their hands, I closed my eyes to go inside and find the psychospiritual issues that were keeping me from a relaxed peace of mind and full happiness in life. I immediately opened my eyes again, saying, "But you don't understand . . ." "Go there now!" was their response. "OK, OK," I said. "I'll go." I shut my eyes. I immediately opened them yet again. "Let me explain it to you this way," I said. "It's like a black hole. Each black hole has an event horizon, the boundary between the area of space where you can still move away from the black hole and the area of space just inside the event horizon, from which escape is impossible, where inevitably, inexorably, eventually you will be sucked down into the black hole itself. I've been to the event horizon of my pain many, many times. It has to do with my mother favoring my older brother and my brother totally rejecting me. I was second best to her, and my brother was no brother to me at all. I've seen that issue many times, from above, and I can tell you about it in great detail. I don't need to go down into the black hole to describe the pain to you. I can tell you all about it." They replied, "Go there now!"

So I went there, spiraling down behind closed eyes, down to the primal experience of being second best to my mother. Immediately, I felt that pain as I had never felt it since the first time I did as a baby, as strongly and as fully as I had originally. I began to cry, feeling wracked by the pain of feeling unloved, unlovable. I opened my eyes, reemerging into the present moment, glaring at my helpers. Through my tears, I cried out: "What do I do with the pain? I told you it would hurt; I told you I could tell you about it! Why did you make me go there and feel this pain? What do I do with the pain?" The Canadian psychiatrist said, "Let me ask you a question: Did you die?"

That moment and that question transformed my life. It was a point I had made to my clients many times: when we are babies, lack of full, grounded, balanced, mature parental love is not only painful, but also scary. We are dependant on our parents for our very lives and if we don't get good parenting, it's not only sad, but also existentially dangerous; we could die of neglect or abuse. Yet as an adult, if we were to be lucky enough to re-experience that lack of healthy, unconditional parental love, it would still be painful—witness my pain when I "went there now"—but . . . it would no longer be dangerous: we can now care for ourselves, even if our parents didn't. That realization is transformative because while pain is awful, it is bearable; we can live through pain, but existential fear cannot be accommodated. As animals, we can never accept or adjust to a fear of death, so we bury and avoid, sometimes for our entire lives, that early, fearful experience. Once we open up the basement door (or have it opened by psychedelics) in a safe and loving therapeutic or sacramental environment, we come to see that while the pain is still there—as strong and as real as the first time we experienced it as a child—the old, locked-in fear is now completely unnecessary, because we can care for ourselves—reparent ourselves now, as adults.

This is what I work on with my clients, and this was what I realized, personally, that day in that tent, with two dear helpers on the Playa at Burning Man. I came to see that I'd been avoiding, yet carrying with me for all those years, my mother's lack of full, unconditional love. It was as if I'd constructed a three-legged chair for my life: if I leaned forward, putting my weight on the right front leg, if, for instance, I was dealing with a shopping chore, I was fine. If I leaned forward, putting my weight on the left front leg, if I was dealing with a business challenge, still fine. Even if I leaned back and put my weight on the right rear leg (the past), thinking about summer camp, I was still fine. But if I put my weight on that phantom left rear leg, if I began to think about my childhood experience of my mother focusing on my older brother, rather than on me, look out! I would become unstable, falling backward into forbidden, hidden, painful, fearful territory, and my default, "neurotic" behavioral strategies would be triggered (in my case, that would mean going for the protection of my intellect, an area that was far away from feelings and with which I was highly successful). Now I felt as if I could accept with compassion my history, my childhood family dynamics, and the personality strategies I adopted as a child. I had the fourth leg of my chair available to me, because the primal fear was gone. That part of my life, though painful, is now readily available to me. I am whole.

With this realization in my heart and mind, I immediately took responsibility for my childhood (for my inner child). Later that day, before the Burn, I went out to a remarkable structure on the Playa called the Temple of Forgiveness. At the beginning of the week, someone said, "Have you been to the Temple of Forgiveness? I cried so much . . ." I thought, "That's pretty emotional, no?" A couple of days later, another person made the same comment: "Have you been to the Temple of Forgiveness yet? I cried . . . " I thought, "Hmm. I wonder what's up with that?" When a third person later made the same comment, I knew I had to visit the temple and that I would cry too.

The Temple of Forgiveness was a three-story wooden structure, and at the Playa level, every square inch was covered with notes, photographs, and penned graffiti, all referring to the deepest relationship and personal concerns, and all expressing or requesting forgiveness. So you might see a piece of paper with the words, "Dad, You abused me when I was defenseless. I forgive you. —Joe," or a photograph of a small child with the inscription "Peter, 2/3/2001–9/5/2006. We love you." The entire first floor—every available space in the temple—was completely filled with heartfelt, gut-wrenching, soul-awakening communications to others who weren't there.

After my guided experience, I, too, had some forgiving to do. I went out to the temple, walking slowly and reading. I cried freely behind my ever-present dust goggles and face mask as I felt the pain and empathy on the walls. I didn't feel ready to write my words yet, so after an hour or so, I left, freshened up, and went out to see the Burning of the Man. The actual Burn is a spectacular event, wildly explosive, with flames, fireworks, jet fuel, and sparks, all witnessed by a writhing crowd of glow-stick and Day-Glo-lit revelers, bodies becostumed, eyes agog and mouths agape, being blown away—sometimes quite literally if they stand too close—by the experience. It's a cross between Hieronymus Bosch's *Garden of Earthly Delights* and the rave scene in the final film in the Matrix trilogy (*Matrix: Revolutions*). The experience was unlike anything I'd ever experienced in my life—it certainly took my mind off my childhood! After falling asleep (or some facsimile of sleep) relatively early, I awoke Sunday morning filled with the feelings from my facilitated psychedelic experience. As I stepped out of the RV, my roommate asked how it had gone, and I just hugged him and began to cry tears of release for all the years I'd held on to resentment and hurt. I cried for a long time. Finally, I had released enough, and after helping to break down our campsite, went back to the temple.

Immediately I found one of the rare blank spots on the wall and wrote "I forgive you . . ." to my brother. My experience with my mother and his unbrotherly treatment of me were not his fault. He was only four when I was born. I next wrote "I forgive you, Dad" to my father, who I also didn't blame for my experience with my mother. Then I sat there for quite some time, staring at that wall, crying again, trying to find the forgiveness for my mother. Somehow, I couldn't completely let my pain and resentment go. Finally, I wrote "I can forgive you, Mom." *Can forgive* indicated that she was theoretically forgivable, but not yet totally forgiven. I left the temple and went to my final shift at Sanctuary. While I was working, the temple, as is tradition, was burned to the ground, and with it, all the resentments and pain inside.

When I got back to New York, I sent a loving, accepting, and forgiving e-mail to my brother, who responded in kind. I hugged and loved my father freely. Everyone noticed my loving behavior. Yet I still felt distant from my mother. Then I asked her to go for a drive with me, and I once again told her how I'd felt about her treatment of me when I was a child. When, as a child, I'd asked her why she loved my brother more than she loved me, at first she simply said that she didn't, that she loved us both equally. As I continued to ask the question over the years, eventually she said it wasn't that she loved me less, but that I needed her love less than my brother. As we drove through the green September suburbs of Long Island, I said that I had the feeling that if she had to do it all over again, she would act the same way toward me. This time, though, she responded that she understood how she'd made a mistake in raising us and would not do it the same way if she could do it over again. Then she apologized to me.

That apology finalized my transformation. I let it all go. That was several years ago, and the change in my attitude toward my family, and toward me, has remained in force. I am still the same person, but I am accepting of my past without being in its grip. I have released my old pain and resentments and am living my life moving forward emotionally, not looking backward.

I tell my clients that they can do the same thing without the aid of psychedelics, and can do so even if their parents have died. However, I must admit that I have been extraordinarily lucky—blessed—to have had the experiences I've had, when I've had them, and to have my parents around—and receptive—to talk about it.

A REVISED VIEW

So, having had both the transcendent and the cathartic psychedelic experience, which do I prefer and support? The answer, as you might have guessed, is both.

The transcendent approach creates a psychological ecology of love and acceptance, providing (perhaps for the first time) the positive regard, safety, and trust that every baby is programmed to crave. Whether it is through a trip where one can touch the glowing, throbbing orb at the ground of our being or from receiving unconditional positive regard as a client in my office, this bottom-up approach eases fear-based resistance to engaging one's depths.

It must be noted here that this transcendent approach is very similar in impact to that reported with the use of MDMA in psychotherapeutic practice. MDMA (Ecstasy) is not a classic psychedelic: there are few if any visual distortions, and the mental trajectory, although definitely "somewhere else"—in an altered state or on a "trip"—is not scary and doesn't make us question our sanity in the way LSD or even mushrooms can. If psychedelics are being given new credibility with the less-notorious and less-distracting name of *entheogens* (generating the theological inside), then MDMA is frequently referred to as an *entactogen*—a substance that can open your core to being touched, by oneself or others. This opening is accomplished not by a brute-force approach of chemically psychologically holding your face to your truth, whether you like it or not, as the classic psychedelics can sometimes do. Rather, MDMA works by melting (almost miraculously) the defenses that normally accompany any spelunking expedition into the depths of one's psychological catacombs. Removing the defensive assault—the chatter—of the personality enables one to go deeper, with only empathy, not criticism, in one's heart. In fact, some recreational users engage in a practice called *candy flipping,* in which they begin with MDMA to relax one's defenses and open up into a loving state of mind, and then take LSD, which can be more challenging, after they've created a more empathic, accepting mind-set. I understand that some of the medical school–based research will soon be experimenting with this approach.

The first effort must be to approach one's psyche from a transcendent perspective—acceptance over analysis, lovingness over critique, development over healing, releasing over fixing. Once that "glowing, throbbing orb at the ground of our being" has been touched and we

remember our empathy, we can be more open and accepting of catharsis, viewing it not as a scary, painful necessity, but as a loving realignment that enables us to move forward with our lives with relaxed
love, rather than protected hiding. When the tension of propping up
a superficial personality structure, of avoiding the painful truth, is
relaxed—when personality is no longer used as personal armor and
is instead the tool for interfacing with the environment, as it was
always designed to be—only then will our natural process of development reinitiate and unfold on its biologically preprogrammed path
toward maturity and wisdom. When catharsis is made safe, it will be
embraced readily, because catharsis enables us to re-see our formative
history and the process of our personality development through our
current, adult eyes. Since as adults we have the formal (or postfor-
mal) operational cognition to be able to take another's perspective—
for example to have empathy for how one's parents came to develop
the personalities they did, to think about the big-picture perspective
of the larger world and Universe, and to think about the future—we
are able to recontextualize and emotionally reposition our view of the
events of our childhood.

So a perspective of transcendent acceptance can ease the cathartic
process of confronting and releasing old, ineffective-but-unconscious
personality strategies "designed by a two-year-old." This is all well and
good—quite beautiful, actually—but since both my steps, the transcendent getting in touch with the ground of my being, as well as
the cathartic "going there now" of my Burning Man experience, were
mediated by psychedelics, how can I incorporate these lessons into my
clinical practice, since I can't use these substances with my clients?

One thing my subsequent experience as a clinician has shown is that
using the transcendent approach of providing total love and acceptance in
tandem with the cathartic approach (through guided imagery) can provide more lasting personal development than either one will when used
separately.

CONCLUSIONS:
WHAT HAVE WE LEARNED?

In drawing near the end of this book, it's appropriate to ask: Where have we been and what have we concluded? Here is an overview of the thought process and conclusions of this book:

The psycheology approach can lead to transformative developmental change.

Transcendent change touches the soul and reaches forward. Love enables us to open to our true self, the transpersonal ground of our being. Going down to my core, clearing the path of defensive structures, inviting my core to unfurl and grow toward the light—this is how transcendence contributes to change.

Cathartic change removes unconscious chains and releases the past. It's ironic that the same pain and fear from the traumatic experience of hot anger or cool withdrawal that led the child to hide in defensive personality, if experienced as adults, would not lead us to choose repression. Re-experiencing the feared event as an adult, with an adult's ability to shift perspective, to think of the big picture, long term, or simply altruistically, relaxes and releases the nexus of defense devised by the child. While the pain of being improperly loved as a baby is still real, the fear the infant feels is gone in the adult.

Transformative developmental change is possible if we reconceptualize personality in the manner prescribed by psycheology, especially with the help of psychedelic therapy.

Safety—love—is the central issue of infancy. Loving behavior toward the infant is strongly associated with its survival, with being fed and protected. If love is missing, the child will feel fear and discomfort—pain. Neglect—not being parented properly, with love, attention, and support—elicits fear of starvation, potential injury, or ultimately death. Babies are genetically wired, through appearing cute and behaving adorably, to make themselves more loveable (literally, able to be loved) because being loved means an increased likelihood of being cared for, and being cared for improves the likelihood of survival—the sole genetic imperative.

Personality is a strategy devised by a child. Of course, children are simply not developed enough cognitively to respond as an adult might to poor parenting. Young children operate in a world of black and white, without the ability to understand how parents got to be the parents they are or what options children might one day have—or just how limited those options are now. Babies don't even perceive themselves as completely separate from the parents; so negative, stressful parenting can have a direct, defining impact on the infant's emerging sense of emotional self. As the child's personality gels in response to the parental ecology, there are diminishing opportunities for the child's original, true self to unfold, supported, in its own directions.

Our true, original self lies under our personality, in the transpersonal ground of our being, at our core. As babies, our original self attempts to connect successfully and lovingly with the parental ecology, but is in some way rebuffed—through either parental anger or parental coolness, the two sides of the coin of poor parenting. Fearing, ultimately, for its survival if it insists on demanding that its needs be met, or a certain aspect of itself be accepted, the baby represses this part of its original self and replaces it with a personality characteristic formed in response to the parents' needs. The earlier, more-real part of us doesn't go quietly into the basement dungeon. No, locked away, it raps on the pipes, becomes a nuisance, and generally makes itself known by way of symptoms. That's why symptoms are our best friend. They are the surface reflection of the cause of our life's difficulties. If we follow the thread of the feelings associated with the symptoms, downward through our history, we will eventually end with the beginning—how the personality came to mask the true self, the symptoms being the chafing of the organism against this devil's bargain.

Empathy and acceptance—love—for ourselves and our parents, enable us to relax and release the knot or nexus in our psyche, to disidentify with the defensive personality and to reidentify with our core self, to finally complete our childhood. Since personality is a strategy developed by a child, it is unlikely to do well as a strategy for adult identity. As structures of the human mind, the ego or persona evolved to effectively interface with the outside world, not to serve as the locus for our identity, which in an integrated self must include our core. In skewed development, the identity resides in the interface with the parents and the fearful world and is not grounded in the core, fundamental self from which, in mature parenting, it would be encouraged to emerge. When, in adulthood, the personality strategy is shown to be unworkable—one gets fired a third time or a spouse leaves—there is an opportunity to see one's personality development clearly, to disidentify with one's personality and reidentify with one's true, core self. That process entails empathy, compassion, acceptance, and love for oneself and for one's family. It both requires and facilitates the emergence of a mature will.

"Neurosis" is the natural, stepwise unfolding of human maturation. It's not about pathology, but spiritual development. That's why it's such a shame to classify this beautiful developmental process as pathological. The word *neurosis* is a huge part of the problem, as it pathologizes normal developmental struggles. One of the most negative influences on psychological development is the *sick* label itself, which tightens and distorts, keeping people from a natural unfolding and realignment. From this perspective, *healing* takes place only when we get underneath our adult personality. When we rest at the ground of our being, we naturally begin again to unfold according to our perfect, inner template for psychospiritual development.

The desire for change is a reflection of the problem, not of the solution. So, working on yourself or your relationships doesn't work. Rather, the thing to do is to be. Striving for change, working on yourself, running around doing things—these approaches will not achieve change, and they can actually make things worse. The desire for change reflects a feeling of not being good enough as you are right now. A good analogy is of a crawling baby learning to walk. Although we hope—and assume—the baby will one day walk and prefer to walk, we don't pathologize age-appropriate crawling. When the baby is crawling, we love the crawling; later, when the baby starts to walk, even as a toddler, we love the walking too. The desire for growth or maturation reflects a sense of one's need for development. It's not necessary to label the process as pathology. Likewise, the process of maturation is naturally effortless and certainly doesn't benefit from the "helpful" analytical skills of the ego. We shouldn't have to work at natural personal development—just as we can't try hard to fall asleep—and it is counterproductive to work on our relationships. The natural, relaxed gut; our whole, grounded self—mind, body, and soul—will do a much better job at being, at growing, and at unfolding than the conscious, analytical part of us alone, or our personality with all its fault lines, skewings, and hiding places.

Transformative developmental change is possible through an interplay between the transcendent and cathartic approaches. The cathartic "frontal assault" approach to personal development, used by itself, is ineffective as it generates too much resistance. The "bottom-up" method of transcending personality issues by starting from a loving core is effective at reducing defenses. Though transcendence generates insight and love, if used only by itself it sidesteps necessary, fundamental, and oftentimes painful realignment and so frequently does not provide lasting change. Only the interplay between safety through loving acceptance and using that safety for undeniable confrontation with self can produce the conditions necessary for the resolution of childhood issues and the reinitiation of one's developmental progression.

Under appropriate conditions, psychedelic therapy can be a safe and extremely effective tool for facilitating transformative developmental change by enabling us to see ourselves clearly and with love and to fully engage in catharsis. Under the right conditions, psychedelics can assist us in relaxing down into the transpersonal ground of our being, where we are at a place of perfect love and acceptance of others and ourselves. From that perspective, our problems or symptoms are re-seen as poignant developmental challenges. Yet if we only apply palliative love for a moment without addressing the unpleasant source of our adult issues at their childhood root, the change will not be permanent. Our personality strategies will reemerge as soon as the day-to-day pressures of life and relationships trigger our unconscious needs.

Catharsis is the process of bringing the unconscious to conscious awareness, and it need not be violent or scary. Rather, we must use loving, transcendent acceptance—just as we encourage our children to walk by loving their crawling—to ease and make safe the catharsis we must go through to achieve balanced, relaxed, integrated personhood.

Stunted or skewed development can be gotten back on track, but psychedelics are not cognitive development—or spiritual maturity—in a pill. By returning us to our deepest, original, true self, by reminding us of the love that is at the core of us all, by enabling us to relax in that love and to release the dynamic tension of defense that is personality— in those ways, psychedelics, under the right conditions, may reinitiate stunted development or realign skewed development, but they cannot advance us into stages of development for which we have not properly gestated cognitively and experientially.

Psychedelics can trigger understanding; on the other hand, behavior change takes time and, in this culture, is often harder to sustain than we acknowledge. A spiritual experience does not make a spiritual life. In fact, psychedelics alone certainly do not provide an answer to difficulties in personality development. One very important adjunct to the use of psychedelics in psychotherapy is development of a meditation practice. Psychedelic experience is dramatic, flooding one with observations, sensations, feelings, insights, and new perspectives and propelling one's understanding forward a vast distance in a very short time. (This experience can be frightening and trigger dramatic, though generally transient, psychological disturbance. This is why psychedelics must be legal and controlled, so we can establish safe methods and settings for their use.) The dramatic contribution of psychedelics takes time to integrate, and this is where meditation comes into play. As dreams are the fuel of psychoanalysis, so are psychedelics the fuel of meditation. I am not speaking of taking psychedelics while meditating, although some have used mild doses of MDMA as an aid to meditation. Rather, I am describing the practice of many who have periodic psychedelic experiences grounded by the daily practice of meditation. Similarly, some theorists have suggested integrating the psychedelic and psycholytic psychotherapeutic approaches, interspersing occasional large psychedelic trips aimed at provoking transformative spiritual development with monthly, smaller trips, perhaps MDMA trips, and integrating these sessions with ongoing psychotherapy. This has been called the psychedelytic approach.[1]

Transformational developmental change requires a stepwise, dualistic dance. We have discussed integrating the cathartic and transcendent approaches to introspection and personal development, potentially facilitated with psychedelics. We have also discussed integrating psychedelics with meditation and large doses of psychedelics with ongoing smaller doses. Maturing through developmental stages results in reintegration, not homogenization. New stages are not a simple averaging of opposing forces, but the development of an entirely new perspective—a perspective created out of, but not predictable from, the prior dualistic interplay. Developmental stages are not traversed in the deliberate, operant sense of purposive analysis and action on a task; rather, developmental stages are built in nested hierarchy and are always in a process of dynamic interplay. As one seemingly impossible challenge is surmounted, we experience a period of easy forward motion, followed by a new "impossible" wall to leap. The two sides of the dynamo generate energy through their differing strengths, as the poles in a battery do as ions migrate.

There are methods for changing policies and bureaucracies, and we are honor bound to bravely apply them in the pursuit of science, truth, freedom, and change. We are all individuals nested in relationship, nested in family, community, nation, ecology, planet, and, ultimately, the universe. This "citizenship" works best when we participate in a full and loving way, and that includes criticism and change. There are methods to change our society built into the system we have inherited. Some parts change rapidly, particularly those linked to generating wealth; others are hidebound and glacial, particularly those linked to protecting assets. There are tools available for change within the system, for change of the system, and even for creative destruction of the system, and we are honor bound as citizens—and as parents—to identify and learn how to use them.

Having laid out the key lessons of this book, as good global citizens we are compelled to actively apply these findings to improve the world. It's important, too, for us to speculate about the future of psychedelic therapy and policy, and whether the reintegration of psychedelics into Western civilization could provide a rite of passage for our culture as a whole, elevating us to a new, integral level of society.

7

IMPLICATIONS FOR THE FUTURE

Psychedelic research with human subjects has been under way again since 1990, and research on psychedelic therapy is now taking place at Harvard, Johns Hopkins, UCLA, NYU, and other institutions worldwide. It's not too early to ask about preliminary findings.

Whether it is MDMA (Ecstasy) for post-traumatic stress disorder, psilocybin for end-of-life anxiety in terminal cancer patients, or ibogaine for heroin addicts, the profile is similar: results are generally positive. While no study has had perfect results, there have been no deaths attributable to taking the study drug during approved research; in fact, there were no undesirable side effects that weren't successfully resolved by the study guide or monitors. To generalize, then, it is fair to say that psychedelic therapy is proving safe when administered in a carefully designed, supportive setting and that the vast majority of subjects, across all studies, report their psychedelic experience as among the most meaningful and positive events of their lives.

More specifically, confirmation appears to be emerging of a tantalizing finding that was just being validated as the earlier phase of research was shut down in the mid-1970s: subjects who showed strong positive results on the outcome variable are more likely to have had a "peak," "integrative," or "religious" experience during the study. It's fascinating to speculate about how the medical community, science, and society in general will respond to the fact that it is a peak or spiritual experience that is doing the healing. While it's true that the body's whole, endogenous systems always do the actual healing, in psychedelic medicine that mediation process is starkly apparent to all. Will we be able to reincorporate a neoanimistic worldview into our hard sciences? We will, if quantum mechnanics is an indicator!

Psychedelics are a catalyzing issue. Although they occupy only a small portion of the cultural mindshare today, over time their reintegration into psychiatry will have an enormous, transformative effect on society as a whole. Psychedelics have the potential to bring science and spirituality into realignment and return us to our healthiest psychospiritual roots. The clinical work under way today is just the beginning; very soon the data will be in, and science will have to accommodate the paradigm-busting impact that psychedelics will have on our view of reality—of healing and medicine, of causation and spirituality. We are trying to accommodate a neotribal perspective that shatters modernity's self-satisfied Cartesian rationale for our planetary split-personality disorder and, in the process, reintegrate and resacralize our lives.

It's almost as if society were surreptitiously slipped a dose of LSD in the 1960s, which society initially enjoyed, but by the time the late '60s rolled around, with Altamont and all those hard drugs, society started to have a bummer, screaming "BAD! Psychedelics are BAD! I don't ever, ever, ever want to take psychedelics again! Neither can you! BAD!" Yet it's been quite a while, and we've been working on society, talking gently, showing the research results, and now society is trying again. Only this time, society is older and wiser, having become quite world-weary about the dangers of psychedelics as expounded by Art Linkletter and any of a number of virtually interchangeable, dour, ill-informed heads of the National Institute on Drug Abuse. So far, this time society seems to be having a good trip.

If research results like the ones I've described continue to come in, and I believe they will, then two changes must surely be made. The first change—that of training psychedelic clinical research associates with the same psychedelic drug they will be giving to their subjects—is already under way, with a Multidisciplinary Association for Psychedelic

Studies protocol for the active training of clinical researchers having just received preliminary approval.

The second change necessary is in the scheduling status of the psychedelics, in particular psilocybin and MDMA. Currently, all the most useful psychedelics are assigned to Schedule I, creating enormous difficulties for the conduct of research. In addition, this farcical situation erodes our ethical landscape, since in order to keep these drugs in Schedule I, the government legally has had to claim that none of the psychedelics have any medical value, a sham position that at the very least, given the fascinating nature of psychedelics, their history, and their potential, deserves vigorous, rigorous reevaluation.

THE CATALYTIC ROLE OF PSYCHEDELICS IN THE EMERGENCE OF AN INTEGRAL SOCIETY

Despite the importance of the clinical research for the use of psychedelics as medicine, the true extent of the impact of psychedelics on society will be felt on the basis of their status as a religious sacrament.

For years, the courts had been applying the American Indian Religious Freedom Act to allow off-reservation peyote possession, but in 1990, the government successfully argued that a Native American defendant's possession of peyote off the reservation was a public health danger that took priority over his First Amendment religious freedoms. Laws that curtail religious freedom for obscure 150-person religions can also be used to curtail religious freedom for large, mainstream religious denominations, so when Congress was inundated by protests from concerned traditional churches, they complained to their colleagues at the Supreme Court. In response, the justices in essence replied that their hands were tied; that the law, as written, simply provided a low hurdle for the government to claim a compelling public interest in restricting religious freedom. In response, Congress soon passed the Religious Freedom Restoration Act of 1993, which places a very strict burden of compelling public need on the government if it wants to restrict the religious freedom of one of its citizens.

One of the results of this strengthening of religious freedom was the recent success of the 130-person U.S. branch of the 10,000-person-strong UDV. The UDV and a similar group, the Santo Daime, have both recently won landmark victories protecting their right to practice their now still-small U.S. religion.

Because visionary psychedelic plants have played such a prominent role in the religious lives of their societies, because prestigious medical schools are conducting research on the therapeutic use of psychedelics (and that research is going well), and because psychedelics have been an issue of religious freedom, I believe psychedelics are playing an axial role—facilitating a fundamental turning point—in our cultural evolution. Psychedelics are playing this axial role for several reasons: they offer a clear, balanced, positive perspective on reality, both intrapsychically and at the societal level; they facilitate a connection to the psychological and the spiritual within; they loosen and deconstruct mind-set, thus facilitating change; and importantly, psychedelics straddle the tribal and the modern worlds. Psychedelics can help us reconfigure from the debacle of industrial modernism and nihilistic postmodernism into an integral society that synergistically combines tribal holism, Western science, and worldwide connectivity, with loving, dharmic, altruism, to become one sustainable planet.

As mentioned above, psychedelic chemicals in the form of visionary plants have been a core feature of societies worldwide, throughout history—all cultures that had access to a visionary plant used it or abandoned one for another that offered a stronger, more reliable experience (the often-mentioned exception is said to be the Inuit, because there are no visionary plants north of the Arctic circle, although dried *Amanita muscaria* would have been available). Furthermore, psychedelics are so self-evidently powerful that they have never completely lost their hold on the imagination of Western scientists and clergy. Now we are experiencing a psychedelic renaissance in government-approved research, yet we still haven't realigned with an explanatory model for the action of psychedelics beyond that of a biomechanistic drug effect. We can best find this new model in an updated version of the time-honored, tribal perspective—a post-postmodern synthesis of tribal and modern—not their average, but a third, completely new transcendence of this classic opposition. Only this third, neotribal, integral worldview can adequately explain psychedelics—the tribal perspective can no longer do so for the modern mind; the modern, deconstructed, industrial perspective surely cannot encompass the tribal experience of visionary plants.

So is survival found in sacred tribal groundedness or are Western capabilities gained through deconstruction? Yes! Does psychedelic therapy work via the action of a serotonin receptor-site agonist, or by touching the face of God? Yes, again! Is the psychedelic effect a neurological phenomenon or an opening to a Universe of energy? Yes, yes, yes!

Another reason why psychedelics are reintegrating into society right now is the age cohort that has been exerting a Jupiter-like gravitational tug on society since I was a child. I myself am a member of this group, the huge "baby boom" explosion of births in America after World War II, from 1946 to 1964.

Today, Boomers are becoming more interested in nootropics. *Nootropics* (literally "mind turning," also referred to as "smart drugs") are compounds, some available only by prescription, that enhance cognitive performance and should be in much demand as this generation ages. It is already acceptable for physicians, in addition to healing the truly sick person back to feeling OK, to proactively give prescriptions to the healthy for chemicals that can make an OK life much better. Why, then, we might come to ask, is it not acceptable for psychiatrists (or clergy; choose your preferred point of entry) to proactively administer to healthy individuals chemicals that have been shown, repeatedly over thousands of years, to be safe and effective at facilitating change and improving quality of life?

Demographically, the Boomer age cohort is approaching the age of physical decline and death. If enough AARP members ask for more involvement in "that wonderful research those nice young men are conducting, giving the chemical in mushrooms to people who are dying of cancer," then the AARP will support it, clamor for it, fund it, and reimburse for it. I can almost hear an AARP lobbyist barking at Congress to support psychedelic therapy for their aging constituents.*

UNITY "VERSUS" THE FRONTAL LOBES

The frontal lobes of the brain, the seat of our brilliant consciousness—of thought, ideation, intention, the ego—are wildly adaptive, yet represent a "devil's bargain": the mindless serenity of integration in nature (a state many Zen meditators seek to recapture) is exchanged for the thoughtful safety of frontal-lobe analysis. A devil's bargain, yes, but supremely adaptive, as we now dominate nature and occupy every corner of the globe. This was the fruit of the tree of knowledge of good and evil: the first division into light versus darkness, soul versus body, energy versus matter, humans versus nature—the first contrasts that enabled discrimination, analysis, extraction, and distillation.

It is an old story by now, how life started out natural yet brutish, and how we evolved adaptations to help us survive. The story of life continues today, as the very traits and brain functions that enabled us to excel thus far are now proving counteradaptive in the form of pollution, extinctions, cancer, obesity, overcrowding, competition and egocentrism, war, addiction to money and material possessions, mechanization, and social alienation.[1] Will we adapt fast enough to see that it is no longer discrimination and analysis, but rather unity and empathy on the global scale that would be most adaptive, that would contribute the most to our survival?

How do we heal that rift, transcend the duality between brutish

---

*I also recommend and hope that all you aging Baby Boomers will write psychedelic research into your wills. If you've read this far, you're obviously at least very interested, and psychedelic research is as sincerely good a cause as anyone could find. An excellent place to start your research on this topic is the Multidisciplinary Association for Psychedelic Studies (www.maps.org) and the Heffter Research Institute (www.heffter.org), both of which fund psychedelic research.

nature and alienated modernity? How do we maintain the benefits of dualism—discrimination, analysis, improved adaptability—and yet transcend the struggle of dualism, to be just one, in our lives, in nature, in the universe?

We must power through today's modern alienation from nature, all the way up and around the spiral of human development to an integral, post-postmodern worldview, not slide back down to a premodern state, as Theodore Kaczynski (the Unabomber) and Osama bin Laden would have it. The integral, post-postmodern position is in alignment with the animist tradition, but a full circle and one level up on the spiral of development. The idea is to embrace a neoanimism, this time with our eyes open, fully conscious, Buddhist-style, for a post-postmodern reintegration of animism and higher awareness.[2] This, then, is a worldview that can accommodate shamanic states and quantum mechanics in one truly natural science.[3]

There are many such related dualities—industrial vs. tribal, mechanistic vs. spiritual, superego vs. id, East vs. West—and yet every duality comprises two halves of one whole. When these seeming dualities are viewed as two halves, the whole question can be seen as the true unit of analysis, not solutions A or B. We can take as our example the neologisms from quantum mechanics, used to describe two perspectives on one thing that can't both be right, but are. The best-known such word is *wavicle,* used to capture the ineffable meta nature of light that is alternately "proved" to be a wave and then "proved" to be a particle. The truth is that it depends on the observer's perspective, derived largely from the measuring instruments one uses to observe the light phenomenon.

As with a wavicle, when we are healed of Cartesian duality, humans might best be seen as a mindbody, a thing of intense intrinsic energy, sometimes dubbed spirit, capable of such godlike flights of perfection in thought or art that the distinction between hand, or eye, or brain and spirit becomes petty and incapable of capturing the true integral nature of our wholeness. Psychedelics have the potential to help initiate and facilitate that process.

When we finally bind that rift, between matter and energy, brain and mind, body and spirit, particle and wave, what will our science be like? Our psychotherapies? Our religions? Moreover, what can we do today to help society in that maturation? For one, we as individuals must develop beyond the simplistic dualities of brain chemistry versus spirituality, tribal versus modern, monotheists versus animists, self versus the outside world. We can develop this unitary worldview—and prepare for an integral society—by accommodating the tribal perspective within our own.[4]

AN INTEGRAL APPROACH TO REALITY

Every worldview contains the seeds of its own eventual dethroning, contradictions that will be explained only by the superseding worldview. Today, it is the integral that is supplanting modernity and postmodernity—the dualism of Descartes being replaced by a worldview that accommodates and integrates opposites: of technology and art, self and other, spirit and flesh. We might refer to this integral approach as a poetry science—not the science of poetry or poetry about science, but a higher-order worldview that positions modern, industrial, extractive science within a broader, poetical, undergirding context of cosmology, creativity, spirituality, and community.

This integration of seeming opposites seems counterintuitive only when viewed from a Newtonian perspective. When we think of the cosmic level of the universe as a whole, counterintuitive, non-Newtonian concepts such as the big bang, time dilation, or a "finite yet boundless" universe are now accepted as normal. Likewise, at the subatomic level of quantum mechanics, we accept seemingly counterintuitive behavior (such as matter springing into existence, or particles communicating instantly over great distances) as the new normal. Yet despite this wonderful insight on nature at the extremes of the subatomic and the cosmic, we still insist that at the human scale, reality is linear, logical, predictable, and mechanistic.

An integral science* that can theorize alternate universes can (and must) also accommodate alternate ways to understand living on Earth. How do states of mind differ from the action of neurotransmitters—and how do both differ from spirituality? It is from an integral perspective that we can finally see that even at the human scale, reality is not fundamentally Newtonian. This integral, human-scale perspective is more consistent with the perspectives of quantum mechanics, relativity, and cosmology that supplanted Newton.[5]

This perspective is based on a nondual, natural philosophy that sees the universe at times as counterintuitive, but never supernatural. We must also apply that idea to viewing the mind: nothing supernatural, just complex and holistic with emergent properties, such as intelligence and consciousness or self-awareness. The same argument can be applied to the universe as a whole: it is emergent—so what some refer to as "miraculous" is still a fully natural gestalt process. The seemingly miraculous or supernatural is just the nature of the universe itself—the whole-is-greater-than-the-sum-of-the-parts gestalt process fully in effect.[6]

This is a holistic, spiritual perspective, but also a scientific one. The integral worldview must successively pass through both spiritual and scientific sieves to reveal its fundamental convergent validity. This requires a holistic approach high enough in perspective to recontextualize and with broad enough inclusiveness to embrace the range of what we've been referring to as the "spiritual."[7]

Many thinkers describe a complex universe, alive at essence, fundamentally, with consciousness (and, ultimately, love) as an emergent property of this complexity.[8] A poetry science sees global mind as the emergent property of life on Earth, spiritual wisdom as simply the fully blossomed end point of normal human development, and the planet as a Gaian organism, embedded in a Gaian universe—and sees all this

---

*An integral science is post-postmodern. That is, after the extractive, power orientation of modernity, after the existential void of postmodern deconstruction, we are now moving toward an integral approach to reality, one that integrates seeming opposites—such as tribal and scientific—and makes us whole again.

not as supernatural, but simply as the normal state of nature.[9]

Over the course of my personal and professional development, I have observed three different perspectives on psychospiritual development:

1. A material view of visionary plants as containing psychoactive chemicals, often extracted or re-created in a laboratory as pharmaceutical drugs, that are seen to interact with endogenous neurotransmitter receptor sites. From this perspective on our personal (and societal) development process, we are conceptually, experientially, and phenomenologically separate from our true self and from everyone else's true self, or soul.

2. A psychological perspective oriented toward healing medical "pathology." In this second perspective, we connect with our true underlying self to provide love for our process of personal development, but we still feeling separate from others—feeling empathy and compassion for our inner child, yet still cursing the person in the car in front of us who cuts us off on the highway on the way to our job caring for the sick.

3. A spiritual view of us as incarnated energy, best conceptualized as love or care for others. In this third perspective, we are finally connected to both our true self and to that of all others. Our personality has become transparent and is no longer calling us, distracting us from our underlying true nature. We see the fundamental unity of reality, of all souls, and radiate spiritual love for everyone and everything.

There have been important tools that have helped me to see these perspectives: psychedelics such as psilocybin and the Mother Vine ayahuasca that open the heart and illuminate the soul; ayurvedic and tantric philosophy; guided visualization techniques; and meditation and yoga, each of which I have found to be effective, nonpsychedelic practices for experiencing transcendence and catharsis in the loving balance so crucial to transformative psychospiritual development.

My fervent hope is that by reading this book, you have been brought along on the path of my own journey in such a way as to better understand and release your own personality, to reindentify with your own true, underlying self—your soul—and that your own life journey will now be clearer, facilitated by, and bathed in, the love of self and others that I believe to be our truest nature.

EPILOGUE

In this book, I've discussed the clinical and ultimately the societal implications of the promising new research on the clinical use of psychedelics. Many people have been helped dramatically by psychedelic therapy—the dying, substance abusers, couples in trouble, sufferers from cluster headaches, victims of post-traumatic stress disorder, those in need of psychospiritual development, and many others.

It is true that the research conducted in the 1950s and 1960s had significant methodological flaws, for example, a dearth of control groups and in many cases the uneven application of care and attention, that contaminate our ability to draw airtight inferences from that earlier, suggestive data. Yet we have learned much in this field over the decades, and in contrast to earlier studies, contemporary designs effectively respond to potential threats to validity, and the methodology of the current research is routinely excellent. A good example of improved contemporary methodology may be found in the impeccable design of Griffiths's recent study of psilocybin's ability to generate mystical-type experiences in normal subjects, which caused even skeptical, longtime drug warriors to praise the study as well as its findings.[1]

Beyond the issue of the clinical applications and study design of psychedelic research, enormous issues of personal freedom are at stake. Researchers require academic freedom to choose the focus of their research and funding to support it; the clergy must defend the right of us all to define our own spirituality, including their own right to be trained with these remarkable spiritual tools; clinicians are ethically expected to provide their patients with the most effective treatments available and patients have the right to receive that state-of-the-art treatment; and individuals should be able to freely experience rites of passage. Yet all are barred from doing so for political, ultimately fear-based reasons. As discussed above, there are tribal roots to these policy issues. Humans seem to have the need and propensity to go through rites of passage: a deconstruction of our current personalities, followed by—with the guidance and the help of our communities—a reconstruction of personality at the next new level, from birth to child, to youth, marriage, parenting, elder, to deathbed.

These needs are still with us. The rave phenomenon is a good contemporary example. Young people are re-creating tribal rites of passage, but without explicit community support and without knowledge of the hard-won safety and efficacy guidelines that evolved over thousands of years in the tribal context. Controlling these substances can have a pivotal impact on our internal freedom, for example, to pursue unpopular meditative traditions.[2] (It is encouraging to note that in a February 2006 United States Supreme Court ruling on a pretrial motion, the UDV church won the preliminary right to use ayahuasca in the United States, and in Oregon in 2009, the Santo Daime finally won a clear victory and the right to use ayahuasca in their ritual.[3]) We need a new policy on psychedelics to match our emergent, integral worldview:

- a rational, objective, systematic policy-making process;
- a less restrictive rescheduling of psychedelics; and
- government funding for approved clinical psychedelic research.

It is crucially important that challenging, new psychopharmacological research be approved *and* funded. How are we going to develop new drugs if we don't enable the psychopharmacologists to conduct their research, including the appropriate application of self-experimentation? To fulfill our responsibility as citizens most effectively, we need to follow where the scientific research takes us, bounded by our humanity, regardless of the political environment. In the current environment for psychedelic research, we are only partially functional: after a very detailed review process, we are seeing psychedelic research protocols eventually gain government approval, but few protocols receive funding from that same government unless they are researching some aspect of drug abuse.[4]

Even so, there is nothing more American than psychedelics, for this is a policy issue that has everything to do with individual freedom, religious freedom, and personal well-being. As a catalyst for debate on topics such as scientific and individual freedom versus government control, psychedelics evoke "life, liberty, and the pursuit of happiness" at its most fundamental, along with a strong dollop of "truth, justice, and the American way" mixed in as well!

Furthermore, there's nothing more democratic than policy research in the service of the greater good.[5] With all the information that's readily available to us now, especially with the widespread emergence of the Internet, it is inevitable that information about the clinical use of psychedelics will continue to diffuse into the public arena and that applications with valid results will ultimately be adopted.

A new perspective on psychedelic research and practice does seem to be emerging today in public policy. If policies and bureaucracies are changing, it may be directly attributable to the decentralization of information and power created by global Internet and wireless telecommunication. These technologies that connect people with people and people with information—and the resultant infocopia of abundant, diverse, and ubiquitous information—are the engines that can enable government to finally fulfill the most far-reaching implications of our Declaration of Independence and Constitution: representational government; fact-based, transparent decision making; governance through innovation, evaluation, and change; intramural cooperation; constituency involvement; and similar democratic promises that can be fulfilled by new technology. In concert with modern techniques for policy change (see appendix I: How to Put Science into Action to Change the

World), this global information infrastructure is providing the psychedelic community with the perfect vehicle to finally drive a transformation of public policy.[6] These changes will not come easily, but the decentralized, virtual government *is* coming—because it can empower people and because it makes economic sense.

Psychedelic researchers and advocates are in a unique and pivotal historical position to influence new government policy through fact-based change. This is an opportunity to open our society to a range of new values, to realign with fact-based policymaking and with serving citizens, and to redefine the role of government away from business, ultimately changing the entire policy-making process.

Bravery has played an enormous role over the history of psychedelic research. Many of the researchers we've discussed have displayed great courage in dealing with psychedelics in their personal as well as in their professional lives. Undoubtedly, there will be a continued need for political bravery, as we are all obliged as citizens to take the actions necessary to move forward this process of rational, evidence-based decision making and change.[7]

We all want to forge a broader, more inclusive, yet still rational view of reality, one that is discriminating among ideas, flexible to change, reasoned in assessment, and systematic in perspective. Our ultimate goal is a more curious, open, accepting viewpoint toward the future—and the present moment—of our development.

Appendix I

HOW TO PUT SCIENCE INTO ACTION TO CHANGE THE WORLD

WORK TO CHANGE THE DRUG LAWS

There are several reasons to change U.S. drug laws. First and most important is that the current drug laws are not based on facts. There are only political reasons, for example, for keeping cannabis in the same category as heroin (or placing heroin there for all purposes, as it is quite useful in easing intractable pain in the dying). This political influence poisons the entire enterprise with a nod-and-a-wink attitude toward the scientific facts. Unfortunately, it is considered appropriate, or at least politically expedient and therefore acceptable, to regulate drugs in this absurd manner.

Furthermore, as mentioned above, in addition to marijuana, essentially all psychedelics have been assigned to Schedule I, the most tightly controlled category, reserved only for drugs that (1) have no medical value, (2) have a high likelihood of abuse, and (3) cannot be administered safely, even by a physician.

This means that academic and scholarly research with psychedelics is very difficult, due to the number of approvals required to use these fascinating, promising agents. In important ways, this also impinges on our religious freedom. I wonder which group will be the test case for the religious freedom to simply practice one's faith without government interference. I wonder how the government would demonstrate a compelling state interest in restricting citizens' exercise of their self-avowed spiritual practice, when the primary dangers are caused by the government making these substances illegal in the first place (which leads to uncertainties in purity and dose), by ignorance (associated with overuse and social stigma), or by behaviors that are already illegal (such as driving while under the influence). Beyond First Amendment arguments, there lies the simple common-sense logic that the punishment shouldn't cause more harm than the crime, which clearly occurs when someone is jailed—taken away from family and gainful, taxable employment—for a primarily victimless crime.

CHANGING PSYCHEDELIC POLICIES AND BUREAUCRACIES

The postmodern, integral, neoanimist perspective presented in this book both results in and requires the changing of society. It's one thing to point to the need to midwife an integral society; it's quite another to go through that labor.[1] Research and practice in the fields of research utilization, change management, knowledge transfer, strategic planning, and the diffusion and implementation of innovations form both the basis and the bias for the analyses and suggestions outlined below.[2] The assumption here is that drug-policy change is a matter of bureaucratic resistance as well as of law[3]; that the politics of drug policy quite often turn on public relations and public education[4]; and that the parsimony of effective practice has honed a set of tools that can be used to change the process of making policies about psychedelics, and thus lead to innovative clinical practices.[5]

Simply put, the body of psychedelic research represents one of the most egregious examples extant of a failure to translate research findings into policy and practice. As such, a conscious effort to understand and influence the dynamics of the policy-making process should improve the utilization of the results of psychedelic research. What follow, then, are some guidelines for putting our money where our mouths are—that is, for translating our insights on policy and practice into effective action and concrete change.

The Policy-Change Process

Policy change is a process, running from initial *awareness* through *interest, evaluation,* and *trial* to ultimate *adoption* of a proposed policy innovation.

To change policy it is important to apply different levers at different points in this process.[6]

As a human process, policy change is strongly influenced by communication about the quality of the data, about the costs and benefits and value of the new policy to the people involved, and about larger strategic and market forces.[7] The process of policy change isn't quite predictable, but it is malleable and therefore leveragable.[8] As such, we can enter into a policy change initiative with the recognition that the regulatory climate can be influenced through communication and that the success rate of policy change proposals can be improved.[9]

Something new is happening in the policy research community. An interwoven set of tools for policy change, including advanced management and planning methodologies and technologies, as well as practical experience gained over the past fifty years of drug policy research and analysis, are coming to critical mass.[10] These techniques, in turn, can enable new, technically oriented proponents of psychedelic research and practice to influence public policy as never before.[11]

Today, these powerful new tools—as local as your laptop, as global as the Internet—are enabling activists to lobby regulatory agencies more effectively. Moreover, the same technology that enables significant participation by local interest groups can also enable the decentralization of the public policy-making process as a whole. In effect, decentralized technologies in hardware (e.g., PCs and laptops), software (e.g., social networking, groupware), Internet sites (e.g., MAPS.org, MoveOn.org, even YouTube.com), and wireless networking have a reciprocal, decentralizing effect on the policy-making apparatus and process, ultimately fostering modularization and decentralization in the structure of bureaucratic power.[12] When we decentralize the technology that enables the bureaucracy, the bureaucracy decentralizes to fit the new infrastructure. Then the bureaucracy fits better to the fundamentally decentralized nature of society, facilitating further alignment of the policy-making process with the community it is meant to serve.

Strategic Alignment

Strategic alignment means "tailoring policy change strategies for key government priorities." The psychedelic community cannot have an agenda entirely its own and expect to have an impact on public policy. Even if it is a "good" agenda, such as implementing the results of state-of-the-art drug policy research, if it's not aligned with the power vector of the policy community, it will likely fail.[13] To be effective in this new, fast, distributed environment, we must align our drug strategy with the current momentum of government. For example, psychedelic therapy research targeted toward treating drug addiction or alcoholism will have a better chance of gaining support than a protocol targeted toward the benefits of recreational use. (As is the case with the Chinese martial art form known as tai chi, once we are aligned with the opposition, we can then use its own momentum to change its trajectory.)

Alignment ultimately becomes a question of which leads to greater success in changing policy: competition or partnership? It is basic social Darwinism—over time, partnership brings success to the most people and provides the most positive net outcome for the country.[14] Therefore, before we can change policy, we have to have policy-change objectives that are aligned with the key priorities of senior government officials and commercial stakeholders.

Even so, it is not the alignment that will provide an opening for effective policy change as much as the presence and advocacy of influential key actors involved in the policy-making process. You must be where policy is being formed when it is happening; it is very difficult to implement change when strategizing from an armchair.[15]

A note of caution, however, is in order: an uncritical emphasis on alignment with the priorities of the powerful can lead to co-optation and is less helpful than no alignment at all. In developing strategies for policy change, advocates find success by building relationships with government agencies and professional groups. As relationships of trust develop, friendships and interdependencies emerge. This is natural, but potentially leads to bias, and so again, care must be taken not to be co-opted by the opposition.[16]

What is the most effective role of the psychedelic community in changing the drug-policy bureaucracy? Partnership. Given the skills required and power matrix involved, the only way for drug-policy change advocates to be effective *and* the only way for a government-policy change effort to succeed is through partnerships. How are we doing on this goal? Results have been mixed. While psychedelic professionals recognize political compromise as crucial to bureaucratic change, many are less than thrilled with the idea of aligning with a set of monolithic government agencies in the process. Nonetheless, while policy-change projects generally *are* run by regulatory agencies and executive or legislative committees, the public interest is so fundamental a consideration in changing drug policy that change agents and advocacy groups inevitably also play a large role.[17]

Psychedelic advocacy groups would seem a natural choice as partners—with psychedelic research and practice supporters among staff in regulatory agencies and legislatures—in a policy change effort.[18] Over the years, effective advocacy groups have honed the skills required for successful policy-change efforts: collaborative focus, process analysis and system design skills, change-management savvy, and teamwork. (The Multidisciplinary Association for Psychedelic Studies and the Council on Spiritual Practices are case studies in partnership with sometimes opposing or recalcitrant institutional "partners.") Interestingly, role models for psychedelic advocacy groups include conservative religious groups, which have become enormously influential in recent years in large part due to their leveraging of marketing and media tools.

Levers of Change

When the advocacy group or change agent has the skill set, what resources should they access? Central among these resources are the change-management levers: *research, people,* and *context.* Each one is necessary, but none is sufficient on its own to ensure change. The research data must be valid and reliable,[19] but must also be relevant to the needs of key actors in various constituency groups.[20] In addition, the larger political, economic, and cultural forces that make up the strategic context in which the government bureaucracy operates must all be addressed. Paying attention to these three interdependent variables—research, people, and context—can improve the odds of a successful bureaucratic or policy-change effort.[21, 22]

The Research Data

The quality of the research design and resultant data gathered is the necessary foundation of success in the dissemination and application of policy research, including efforts at data-based organizational change. If the research data are not valid and reliable, no subsequent efforts at implementation and change will, or should, succeed. Good research data come in many varieties, however, including biochemical analysis of blood and medical imaging of psychedelic subjects under varying conditions, clinical observations by experimenters, content analysis of subject accounts or of creative output such as artwork, questionnaires and surveys assessing attitudes and opinions of subjects and the public, and demographic analysis of population data.[23] There is a preferred method of analysis for each of these types of data, from the statistical to the qualitative, as well as criteria for significance.[24] While quantitative data enable precise analysis, qualitative forms of data provide breadth and context that can substantially improve the validity of our inferences, our logic, and our generalizations from the data.[25]

The People in the Organization

Even though a relevant, data-based proposal for change in a policy or bureaucracy is the necessary starting point, facts are by no means sufficient to ensure change. Due to human anxiety over change or loss of power and esteem, resistance is to be expected. Without organizational support, even a policy proposal based on valid and reliable research data is unlikely to be implemented.[26]

There are two sets of people levers, because in most organizational settings there are two influential interest groups. One group comprises the decision makers—the agency heads, key legislators, influential lobbyists, and top pharmaceutical industry executives, for example—who, after study, advice, and arm-twisting, will be the ones to develop the consensus on whether to introduce a new drug policy to the nation, or even to revamp the drug-policy-making apparatus. Yet decisions made by fiat from on high in a bureaucracy have a very poor track record of successful implementation. This is due to the second interest group—the implementers—who actually craft and implement the new policies. While the president can always say, "We're going to do it!" the policy wonks and bureaucratic rank and file of each interest group can still dramatically alter or even kill a project if they're not on board. To improve the likelihood of change in bureaucracies and policies, the needs of both key interest groups must be addressed.[27]

Decision makers and implementers tend to be motivated by different issues.[28] In large corporations, such as pharmaceutical firms, decision makers tend to be motivated by quantifiable proof that the product will perform safely and effectively and garner a large market share, thus contributing to the organization's bottom line and so to their annual bonus (and job security). Staff implementers, on the other hand, tend to be motivated more by the effect of any resultant changes in procedure on their span of control and quality of worklife. Both groups want assurance that a decision to support psychedelic research and practice won't blow up in their face politically, compromising their careers.

In order to avoid irrelevance in the eyes of decision makers and the "not-invented-here" syndrome among staff, change agents must address each interest group's unique priorities. In fostering policy change among top decision makers, we must manage decision-maker concerns about safety, efficacy, and economic viability. In fostering policy change among staff, we must safeguard a sense of ownership by sharing decision-making authority and building trust relationships. We must provide political air cover for both groups through the liberal application of hard data and a flexible, strategic perspective on real politics (which I will discuss next).[29]

The Strategic Context

Even with valid and reliable policy research data in hand, attending to interest group issues is a necessary but still insufficient condition to effect data-based policy innovation and bureaucratic change. The third and final lever of policy change is the *strategic context*—the political, cultural, and economic big-picture issues that constrain or facilitate change.[30] These are issues of market trends for products based on psychedelics, the political climate, the economy, and community and public-relations concerns, all of which can derail an innovative policy if not addressed.*

---

*One particularly determinant—and particularly thorny—issue is that of the way we finance our political campaigns. It is clear that politics follows the golden rule of business: "Whoever makes the gold, makes the rules." In other words, our politicians serve those who finance their campaigns, and so, their career continuity. If we are to sway public policy, we must follow the admonition of Watergate's Deep Throat and "follow the money." We must either reform campaign finance rules, or use them full out to the advantage of our cause.

It is only when all three levers of change—*research, people,* and *context*—have been considered that we have both the necessary and the sufficient conditions to facilitate data-based change in policy and bureaucracy. Understanding the change process, aligning with policy priorities, and skillfully using all available levers of change are all essential if we are to influence policies and bureaucracies. Even so, without changing our worldview—and our personal values and priorities—we will be unsuccessful in effecting change in the outside world.

PRACTICE "RIGHT ACTION": BUDDHISM AND PSYCHEDELICS POLICY

As part of changing our personal values and priorieties, it is helpful to seek practical guidelines.* All religions provide guidelines for right (or righteous) living—attitudes and behaviors that are likely to lead to a happy life. I have found Buddhist ideas inspirational for my own journey, and below I've included the Buddhist Eightfold Path as an example of this mind-set.

The Noble Eightfold Path of Buddhism

Wisdom

1. *Right view.* Understand things as they are.
2. *Right intention.* Commit to ethical and mental improvement.

Ethical Conduct

3. *Right speech.* Be honest; speak with love; talk only when necessary.
4. *Right action.* Behave in a beneficial way to others and to self.

---

*I am always surprised that more religious adepts and scholars of religion don't embrace the psychedelic research community, either as informed subjects who could help describe and explain what they experience experimentally or as researchers who could develop incisive research protocols based on their knowledge of the hidden terrain of the mind. With increased research supporting psychedelic mysticism, we may see this situation rapidly change.

5. *Right livelihood*. Respect right speech and right action in one's work.

Mental Development

6. *Right effort*. Cultivate the mental energy to abandon unwholesome activities and to increase wholesome ones.
7. *Right mindfulness*. Be aware of the process of conceptualization; actively observe and control the way one thinks.
8. *Right concentration*. Develop one-pointedness of mind through meditation.

The suggested attitudes and behaviors in the Eightfold Path compel us to work hard to protect the vulnerable and to change public policies that are harmful to the general welfare.

Appendix 2

STANDARDS FOR SAFE AND EFFECTIVE PSYCHEDELIC JOURNEYS AND PROCEDURES FOR HANDLING PSYCHEDELIC EMERGENCIES

There are three parts to psychedelic work: preparation, conduct of the session and reintegration, and handling difficult sessions. Below I provide readings and a set of guidelines for each part.

PREPARATION: CREATING A SAFE SPACE FOR PSYCHEDELIC JOURNEYS

Preparation Reading:
General and Background Information about Psychedelics

When it comes to creating a safe space for psychedelics, the more you understand these substances and their background, the more at ease you will be during sessions or when helping others in a session. To this end, I suggest the following readings to begin building your foundation of knowledge.

Psychedelic Drugs Reconsidered, L. Grinspoon and J. Bakalar
This source offers the single best introduction to the facts of psychedelics.
New York: The Lindesmith Center, 1997.
www.drugpolicy.org/library/bookstore/pdrad2.cfm

Shroom: A Cultural History of the Magic Mushroom, **Andy Letcher**
This book offers an extraordinary intellectual achievement in popular scholarly inquiry. It is incisive, skeptical, brilliantly analyzed, and beautifully written by an insider.
New York: HarperCollins, 2007.
www.harpercollins.com/books/9780060828288/Shroom/index.aspx

Pharmacotheon: Entheogenic Drugs, Their Plant Sources and Histories,
J. Ott, foreword by Albert Hofmann
This book offers a more scholarly, in-depth overview of psychedelics.
Kennewick, Wash.: Natural Products Company, 1993.
www.erowid.org/library/review/review_pharmacotheon1.shtml

Storming Heaven: LSD and the American Dream, **Jay Stevens**
This book provides a fun, informative cultural background on America's
drug-induced visionary history (1870s–1966).
New York: Harper and Row, 1988.
www.stormingheaven.com/

"Psychotherapy and Psychedelic Drugs"
This is a listing of seventeen books and articles on the topic compiled by the
"Psychedelic Library," one of the most comprehensive collections of primary
documents in the field.
Published online by the Psychedelic Library.
www.psychedelic-library.org/thermenu.htm

Preparation Guidelines:
Values and Procedures for the Setting

Those creating a psychedelic-friendly event have the responsibility to make it
safe, to the extent that such is possible. The following are the services that,
at a minimum, should be available.

- ▶ Water, a place to recline, and staff members who can shape the setting to the needs of the attendees. While no "treatment" is expected
  or appropriate, it is important for staff to be able to recognize when
  attendees need outside help and when they can safely continue to be
  accommodated in the event environment.

▶ Dosing without the recipient knowing about it or giving permission is like rape—not a gift, not a psychedelic act, and never OK. This value must be actively promoted in the culture of the hosting organization.

▶ The purpose of sitting with attendees in crisis is not to reduce effects, but to create and maintain a safe place where individuals can play out their process without coming into conflict with themselves or others.

▶ While sitting, transference (of fear, of not wanting to get involved, of power, of attraction, and so forth) is inevitable and should be acknowledged, talked about in advance, and managed.

▶ No sexual acting out is permissible, ever.

▶ The community member in crisis deserves discretion and confidentiality.

▶ The community member in crisis shouldn't be left alone.

▶ Sitters should be ready to face difficult times and stay around.

▶ Psychedelic-friendly events should have medical staff on call, but if a safe space is created, they will rarely be necessary.

THE SESSION: GUIDELINES FOR SAFE AND EFFECTIVE PSYCHEDELIC JOURNEYS

Reading and Learning about a Session: Guidelines for Journeys

The following sources are provided as deep background, crucial to the mindful conduct of those helping others in the safe and effective use of psychedelics.

"Guidelines for the Sacramental Use of Empathogenic Substances," by Sophia Adamson

From the Guidelines:

The following guidelines have been compiled from the collective experience of about twenty or thirty therapists who have used these substances in their work, and who have based their methods on observation of hundreds of individual sessions. While there is by no means uniformity of approach among the different practitioners, the guidelines offered here do represent a kind of distillation of methods that have proven their efficacy. Their description here should not in any way be construed as an encouragement to the use of illegal substances. Rather they are applicable to any state of heightened empathic awareness, regardless of how it is generated.

Although the use of MDMA and other drugs of this family occurs statistically most frequently in what might be called a hedonistic or recreational context, with no particular therapeutic or spiritual purpose in mind, these types of sessions will not be discussed here. It is the belief of the present author, and of the therapists and individuals represented in this book, that such recreational use, while probably harmless (certainly less harmful than alcohol or tobacco), does not have the intrinsic interest and healing potential that the guided, intentional, therapeutic, and sacramental use has. The approach will be described under the headings of Preparation and Set, Alchemical Catalysts, Setting and Context, Process and Method in Individual Sessions, Ritual Structure in Group Sessions, and Re-entry and Follow-up Factors.

Published online by MAPS.
www.maps.org/gateway/%5b55%5d181-197.html

"Sitters or Guides," Nicholas Saunders

Provides guidance on choosing a sitter, being a sitter, deciding whom to sit for, preparation, the venue, the session, and afterwards.
Published online by the Council on Spiritual Practices, 1998.
csp.org/nicholas/A59.html

"Code of Ethics for Spiritual Guides," Council on Spiritual Practices

From the Code of Ethics: "Spiritual practices, and especially primary religious practices, carry risks. Therefore, when an individual chooses to practice with the assistance of a guide, both take on special responsibilities." The Council on Spiritual Practices proposes a Code of Ethics covering the following topics, for those who serve as spiritual guides:

- ▸ Intention
- ▸ Serving Society

- ▶ Serving Individuals
- ▶ Competence
- ▶ Integrity
- ▶ Quiet Presence
- ▶ Not for Profit
- ▶ Tolerance
- ▶ Peer Review

Published online by the Council on Spiritual Practices, 2001.
www.csp.org/development/code.html

"Ethical Caring in Psychedelic Work," Kylea Taylor, M.S.

From "Ethical Caring in Psychedelic Work":

> In psychedelic work, the potential is greater for stronger, more subtle, and more complicated transference and countertransference to occur. . . . Steps need to be taken to ensure that if psychedelic research is someday adopted by mainstream science, the job qualifications for sitter will include that he or she has done effective, deep personal work in nonordinary states.

Taylor's excellent article covers the following topics:

- ▶ Quantitative and qualitative differences in ethical psychedelic work
- ▶ The greater need for a safe setting for persons experiencing nonordinary reality
- ▶ The need for an expanded paradigm
- ▶ Personal issues of counter-transference: money, sex, and power

MAPS Newsletter 7, no. 3 (Summer 1997): 26–30.
www.maps.org/news-letters/v07n3/07326tay.html

"Counter-Transference Issues in Psychedelic Psychotherapy," Gary Fisher

From Fisher's article:

> In a 1997 MAPS Bulletin article, Kylea Taylor [see article listing, above] addressed the unique circumstances that arise for the psychedelic psychotherapist (the sitter). She adequately described the special needs of the psychedelic voyager (the client), which need not be repeated here. This note is to further elucidate the counter-transference issues in the

psychedelic therapy setting and to offer some procedural considerations for its effective management.

Fisher's article covers:

- ► Self-acceptance of the sitter
- ► Sitters' meeting before a session
- ► Unexpected therapeutic effect
- ► Resolving counter-transference
- ► A note on schizophrenia

MAPS Bulletin 10, no. 2 (Summer 2000): 4.
www.maps.org/news-letters/v10n2/10204fis.html

"Psychedelic Psychotherapy: The Ethics of Medicine for the Soul," Brian Anderson

From the abstract:

Psychedelic drugs like LSD and MDMA (Ecstasy) are known to have profound psychological effects on people. These substances are now being evaluated in clinical trials in the US as aids to psychotherapy. The use of these substances in Transpersonal Psychology is thought to help patients by inducing spiritual experiences that lead to improved mental health. Some people challenge the claim that authentic spiritual experiences can be induced by drugs and still others question whether spirituality has any place in medicine at all. The potential emergence of the use of psychedelics in medicine calls for a consideration of these and many other concerns.

Penn Bioethics Journal 2, no. 1 (2006): 1–4.
www.maps.org/media/u_penn_3.17.06.pdf

Guidelines for the Session:
Set and Setting, Safety and Efficacy

The following guide for creating a safe psychedelic space is from the work of Jim Fadiman, Ph.D., a psychologist (Harvard, Stanford) and one of the world's foremost scholars of psychedelics. He was an early colleague of Abraham Maslow, Timothy Leary, and Ram Dass at Harvard, and Myron Stolaroff and Willis Harman at Stanford.

Setting

Voyager and Guide

- ▶ A private, safe, comfortable indoor space for the session's duration.
- ▶ Specifically comfortable spots—couches, beds, rugs—for Voyager to lie down, sit down, and hang out in.
- ▶ Soft pillows and blankets available.
- ▶ Music capability: headphones, earbuds, or speakers available in accordance with Voyager's preference.
- ▶ Eyeshades, eye pillows, a folded washcloth or scarf for eyes-closed music listening.
- ▶ Flowers and candles if desired.
- ▶ Water for Voyager and Guide.
- ▶ Adequate restroom facilities.
- ▶ Electronic devices (including phones) are silenced or turned off.
- ▶ Have otherwise minimized likelihood of external interruptions.
- ▶ Have art materials, journals, and other creative tools available for Voyager's use, if desired.
- ▶ Family photographs, a mirror, artistic objects, flowers, and other beautiful natural or manmade objects available.
- ▶ Agree on whether outdoors is safely accessible for latter part of session.

Voyager

- ▶ Adequately and comfortably dressed and have warm layers available.
- ▶ Have consulted with Guide on music, and, if desired, have provided Guide with specific musical requests and selections.

Guide

- ▶ Feel good about the space and overall setting.
- ▶ Have provided for personal food, drink, and other needs for duration of session.
- ▶ Have consulted with Voyager on music.
- ▶ Have appropriate music available for different phases of session, e.g., have wordless music available for first 2–3 hours, and so forth.

Session

Voyager and Guide

▸ Prepared, positive, and overall ready for duration of coming session.

▸ Have no sudden intense forebodings or misgivings about going forward with imminent session.

▸ Create intentional, sacred space as entheogen is administered.

▸ Agree to keep unnecessary conversation to a minimum.

▸ An appropriate sitter is available to care for the Voyager at the end of the session and after the session.

Voyager

▸ Have eaten lightly or not at all before session.

▸ Feeling physically well (or well enough) to go forward with session.

▸ Prepared to take guidance and receive assistance from the Guide during the session.

▸ Prepared to lie down, listen to music, observe breathing and pay attention to any sensations in the body.

▸ Prepared to let go of expectations about session, let go of personal concerns about relationships, personal issues, and habits.

▸ Prepared to let go of each experience, feeling, or visual event as it occurs.

▸ Prepared to let go of my personal identity and allow physical boundaries to dissolve.

▸ Prepared to experience and deepen my awareness of other dimensions of reality.

▸ Will ask for Guide's help, assistance, or feedback whenever desired. Will trust Guide's directions.

▸ Prepared to reintegrate toward the end of the session.

Guide

▸ Prepared to give Voyager specific necessary assistance and guidance, such as gentle touch and the suggestion to breathe deeply.

▸ Prepared to assist Voyager in getting to and going to the bathroom.

▶ Prepared to hold Voyager's hand, etc.

▶ Remember to let Voyager know you are leaving, and have come back, if need to briefly leave to use bathroom or otherwise.

▶ Also prepared to go with overall flow, to trust Voyager's instincts, and to accommodate Voyager's stated desires when reasonable and possible.

▶ Will take no consciousness-altering drugs before or during the session.

▶ Prepared to experience and appropriately deal with any "contact high."

▶ Will not be sexual, even if asked.

▶ Will validate what Voyager sees and experiences by rephrasing or summarizing it in simple language.

▶ Prepared to invite Voyager to go deeper by saying phrases like, "Yes! That's good. Would you like to know more?"

▶ Prepared to show Voyager personal photographs one by one.

▶ Prepared to make electronic recordings or take notes at Voyager's request.

DEALING WITH PSYCHEDELIC EMERGENCIES (OR SPIRITUAL EMERGENCE)

Reading about Difficult Psychedelic Experiences and Spiritual Emergenc(y)

Since psychedelics are still illegal, much of the safety net usually provided by society for the use of medicines or engagement in other potentially dangerous behaviors (such as driving, sky diving, SCUBA diving, and the like) are not in place. Even so, millions of citizens take psychedelics and so it is the most responsible citizenship to try to reduce the harm that might occur from the use of unregulated substances. These guidelines will help all of us improve the outcome of a difficult psychedelic experience in others we might encounter.

People who may be involved in responding to a psychedelic emergency should be familiar with several resources.

Working with Difficult Psychedelic Experiences, J. Davies
This 20-minute educational video is a practical introduction to the principles of psychedelic therapy. It teaches psychedelic drug users how to minimize psychological risks and explore the therapeutic applications of psychedelics. Narrated by Donna Dryer, M.D., the video demonstrates examples of when and how to help a friend, peer, or loved one make the most out of a difficult experience with psychedelics.
Produced by Bricolage Media and MAPS.
www.maps.org/wwpe_vid/

**"How to Treat Difficult Psychedelic Experiences: A Manual,"
Anonymous**
This manual was written by a psychedelic therapist for the use of lay volunteers who are helping those undergoing difficult psychedelic experiences.
www.maps.org/ritesofpassage/anonther.html

**"A Model for Working with Psychedelic Crises at Concerts and Events,"
B. Doyle**
This is a MAPS article on the Serenity Tent at the Hookahville music festival, at which volunteers worked alongside a medical team to help concertgoers work through difficult experiences.
Maps Bulletin 11, no. 2 (2001).
www.maps.org/ritesofpassage/model_working_with_psychedelic_crises_concerts_events.html

**"Crisis Intervention in Situations Related to Unsupervised Use of
Psychedelics," S. Grof**
This piece offers an experienced psychedelic therapist's perspective on working with difficult psychedelic experiences.
Appendix I, *LSD Psychotherapy.* Alameda, Calif.: Hunter House, 1980, 1994.
www.psychedelic-library.org/grof2.htm

**"Psychedelic Crisis FAQ: Helping Someone through a Bad Trip, Psychic
Crisis, or Spiritual Crisis," Erowid**
This document offers lots of concrete suggestions for helping someone undergoing a difficult psychedelic experience. It also helps in determining whether a

person's condition is critical and requires medical intervention, or if it should be treated as a medically stable psychedelic crisis.

Published online by Erowid. Version 2.1 (August 1, 2005). www.erowid.org/psychoactives/faqs/psychedelic_crisis_faq.shtml

Guidelines for Helping with a Difficult Psychedelic Experience or Spiritual Emergenc(y)

Here is an especially useful excerpt from the Erowid "Psychedelic Crisis FAQ: Helping Someone through a Bad Trip, Psychic Crisis, or Spiritual Crisis":

- ▸ If someone seems to be having a hard time, gently ask them if they would like someone to sit with them. If it seems disturbing to them to have someone sitting with them, have someone nearby keep an eye on them unobtrusively.

- ▸ Relate to them in the space they are in. Oftentimes, the thing which isolates people and creates a sense of paranoia or loss is that they are *so far out* of normal awareness that people are trying hard to ground them. Start off instead by trying to just be there for them. Try to see the world through their eyes.

- ▸ What different ways can you change setting (noise level, temperature, outside vs. inside, etc.)? A party/rave/concert setting can aggravate a person's state of mind. Consider finding the quietest place if it seems like it will help (taking cues from the experiencer), and ask people to not crowd around. Reassure them the situation is under control, noting those who offer help in case help is needed later.

- ▸ How can you minimize risk of emotional or physical harm? Remember your concern for how the person is feeling, not concern for the situation (as in "oh my gawd, we've got to do something").

- ▸ Paranoia: If the person doesn't want anyone near them, hang back, turn so you aren't staring at them, but keep an eye on them as discretely as possible. Think about what it would feel like to be in a paranoid state, having some stranger (whether you are or not) follow you around and watch you.

▶ What objects/activities/distractions might help the person get through a difficult space (toys, animals, music, etc.)?

▶ No Pressure: Just be with them. Unless there is risk of bodily injury, just make it clear you are there for them if they need anything.

▶ Touch can be very powerful, but it can also be quite violating. In general, don't touch them unless they say it's OK or they touch you first. If it seems like they might need a hug, ask them. If they are beyond verbal communication, try to be very sensitive to any negative reaction to touch. Try to avoid getting pulled into any sexual contact. Often, holding hands is a very effective and non-threatening way to let someone know you are there if they need you.

▶ Intensity can come in cycles or waves. It also can work as a system— a movement through transpersonal spaces that can have a beginning, a middle, and an end. Don't try to push too hard to move it.

▶ Not Forever: If they are connected enough to worry about their sanity, assure them that the state is due to a psychoactive and they will return to their "home" state of mind in time.

▶ Normal Drug-Induced: Tell them they are experiencing the acute effects of a psychoactive (if you know what, tell them) and tell them that it is normal (although uncommon) to go through spiritual crises and they (like thousands before them) will be fine if they relax and let the substance run its course.

▶ Breathe with them. If they are connected enough to be present for assistance, get them to join you in deep, long, full breaths. If they're amenable to it, or really far out and freaking, putting a hand on their belly and saying, "breath from down here," "just keep breathing, you got it," can help.

▶ Relaxing: It can be very very hard to relax in the middle of dying or being pulled apart by demons, but tell them that you are there to make sure nothing happens to their physical body. One of the most important things during really difficult internal processes is to learn to be OK with them happening, to "relax" one's attempt to stop the experience and just let it happen.

- ▶ Getting meditative: Gently suggesting they try to close their eyes and focus inward can sometimes change the course of their experience.
- ▶ Bare feet on the ground: One of the most centering and grounding things to do is to take off shoes and socks and get your feet directly on the hard ground. Be careful of doing this in toe-dangerous surroundings.
- ▶ Eye contact: If the person is not acting paranoid and fearful of you, make sure to include a lot of eye contact.
- ▶ Everything is fine with me: Make it clear that the world may be falling apart for them, but everything is OK with you.
- ▶ Healthy process: Crises are a normal part of the human psychological process and one way to engage them is as a process of healing, not a "problem" to be fixed.
- ▶ The most comforting thing some people have reported helped them during acute experiences is a blanket wrapped around them. We cannot recommend enough having a thick, weighty blanket for emergencies.

RECOMMENDED READING

FAMILY

Between Parent and Child: The Bestselling Classic That Revolutionized Parent-Child Communication, **Hiam G. Ginott**
What children need to individuate with esteem and how to develop a communicative relationship with your child. (New York: Three Rivers Press, 2003.)

Getting the Love You Want: A Guide for Couples, **Harville Hendrix**
Lays out the process of personality formation and how we project childhood needs onto our mates; describes an effective method for waking up and completing your childhood. (New York: Harper Perennial, 1991.)

The Continuum Concept: In Search Of Happiness Lost, **Jean Liedloff**
Generalizations from anthropological fieldwork data on how tribal cultures treat their infants. (Cambridge, Mass.: Da Capo Press, 1986.)

COGNITION AND BRAIN

The Dragons Of Eden: Speculations on the Evolution of Human Intelligence, **Carl Sagan**
How the brain is built upon reptilian and earlier substrates, which manifests in our behavior. (New York: Random House, 1977.)

The Origins of Intellect: Piaget's Theory, **John L. Phillips Jr.**
How cognition matures from birth through adolescence. (San Francisco, Calif.: Freeman, 1969.)

CULTURAL ANTHROPOLOGY

The Denial of Death, **Ernest Becker**
How our sublimation of existential angst results in our great works. (New York: Free Press, 1973.)

Civilization and Its Discontents, **Sigmund Freud**
How and psychoanalytically why civilization arose. (New York: W. W. Norton, 1961.)

The Naked Ape: A Zoologist's Study of the Human Animal, **Desmond Morris**
Our animal nature in body and signs. (New York: McGraw-Hill, 1967.)

Plants of the Gods: Their Sacred Healing and Hallucinogenic Powers, **Richard Evans Schultes and Albert Hofmann**
Survey of the major visionary plants and their shamanic cultures, by the director emeritus of the Harvard Botanical Museum and the Sandoz chemist who discovered LSD-25. (Rochester, Vt.: Inner Traditions, 1992.)

The Wise Wound: Eve's Curse and Everywoman, **Penelope Shuttle and Peter Redgrove**
How women's menstrual cycle is special and wondrously witchlike. How it is revered and tapped in tribal societies and should be now, too. (New York: Richard Marek Publishers, 1978.)

PHILOSOPHY

The Mind of Light, **Sri Aurobindo**
Describes the evolution of consciousness as the purpose of life; tells future direction; includes annotated bibliography. (Whitefish, Mont.: Kessinger Publishing, 2006.)

The Tao of Physics: An Exploration of the Parallels Between Modern Physics and Eastern Mysticism, **Fritjof Capra**
How Eastern philosophy and Western physics are both groping at the same core reality. (Berkeley, Calif.: Shambhala Press, 1975.)

The Systems Approach, **C. West Churchman**
How the world is organized in a nested, hierarchical fashion. (New York: Dell Publishing, 1968.)

Visions of Innocence: Spiritual and Inspirational Experiences of Childhood, **Edward Hoffman**
Dozens of brief verbal reports of spontaneous visionary experiences of small children, often relayed for the first time, decades later, by the now elderly subject. (Berkeley, Calif.: Shambhala Press, 1992.)

The Perennial Philosophy, **Aldous Huxley**
Looking across all religions, Huxley generalizes twenty-seven universal spiritual truths, in twenty-seven very dense chapters. (New York: Harper and Row, 1944.)

The Awakening of Intelligence, **Jiddu Krishnamurti**
Describes how our analytical thinking is counterproductive to our peace of mind, and talks about releasing the perfection inside. Develops the idea of will as our inner, driving force. (New York: Discus, 1976.)

The Future of the Body: Explorations into the Further Evolution of Human Nature, **Michael Murphy**
Encyclopedic overview of all progressive approaches to spiritual/personal development. After a systematic review of techniques for transformative change, Murphy zeroes in on Psychosynthesis, Krishnamurti, and Sri Aurobindo, as the most effective. (Los Angeles, Calif.: Jeremy P. Tarcher, 1992.)

PSYCHEDELICS AND SOCIETY

Psychedelic Drugs Reconsidered, **Lester Grinspoon and James Bakalar**
The best short, accessible overview on plant sources, tribal antecedents, clinical applications, nature of the experience, adverse effects and contraindications, spiritual effects, and legal issues. Includes an extensive annotated bibliography. (New York: The Lindesmith Center, 1997.)

Island, **Aldous Huxley**
Huxley's utopian response to his own dystopia, *Brave New World*. Depicts a society where entheogens are integrated into society and used to facilitate rites of passage. (New York: Harper and Row, 1962.)

Storming Heaven: LSD and the American Dream, **Jay Stevens**
The visionary history of the West in the seventy years from the extraction of mescaline from peyote and its ingestion by Arthur Heffter in 1897, to the "Death of the Hippie" parade in Haight-Ashbury on October 6, 1967. (New York: Harper and Row, 1988.)

ADVANCED TEXTS

Psychotherapy East and West: A Unifying Paradigm, **Swami Ajaya**
Sweeping overview of classical, humanistic, dualistic, and monist perspectives on human nature; direct applications in psychotherapy. (Honesdale, Pa.: Himalayan Institute Press, 1983.)

Essence with the Elixir of Enlightenment: The Diamond Approach to Inner Realization, **Ali Hameed Almaas**
Discussion of monist philosophy, and the proper training for advanced spiritual seekers. (New York: Weiser Books, 1998.)

Psychosynthesis: A Collection of Basic Writings, **Roberto Assagioli**
Discussion of psychosynthesis (a synthesis of Eastern philosophy and Western psychoanalysis) by its founder. (Amherst, Mass.: The Synthesis Center, 2000.)

The Leaven of Love: A Development of the Psychoanalytic Theory and Technique of Sandor Ferenczi, **Izette de Forest**
An overview of the life and philosophy of psychoanalyst Sándor Ferenczi, a believer in direct relationships with patients. (Cambridge, Mass.: Da Capo Press, 1984.)

The Origins of Order: Self-Organization and Selection in Evolution, **Stuart Kauffman**
Why the increase in order and complexity is built into the structure of the universe, which means that the evolution of life and intelligence is inevitable. (New York: Oxford University Press USA, 1993.)

The Ecstatic Imagination: Psychedelic Experiences and the Psychoanalysis of Self-Actualization, **Dan Merkur**
Includes a developmental psychology of advanced seekers. (New York: SUNY Press, 1998.)

Pharmacotheon: Entheogenic Drugs, Their Plant Sources and History, **Jonathan Ott**
Encyclopedic history and reference text for psychedelic substances and culture. (Kennewick, Wash.: Natural Products, 1996.)

Yoga and Psychotherapy: The Evolution of Consciousness, **Swami Rama, Rudolf Ballentine, and Swami Ajaya**
Fundamental ayurvedic, hygienic, health approach to life, personality, meditation, breathing, and psychotherapy. (Honesdale, Pa.: Himalyan Institute Press, 1976.)

Sensitive Chaos: The Creation of Flowing Forms in Water and Air, **Theodor Schwenck**
How the flow of matter reveals the underlying nature of the universe. (New York: Schocken Books, 1976.)

The Rebirth of Nature: The Greening of Science and God, **Rupert Sheldrake**
Why and how we need to resacralize—and dereligify—our modern worldview.
(Rochester, Vt.: Park Street Press, 1992.)

PiHKAL: A Chemical Love Story, **Alexander Shulgin and Ann Shulgin**
Encyclopedic listing of phenylethylamine chemistry, pharmacology, and subjective effects. (Berkeley, Calif.: Transform Press, 1993.)

TiHKAL: The Continuation, **Alexander Shulgin and Ann Shulgin**
Encyclopedic listing of tryptamine chemistry, pharmacology, and subjective effects. (Berkeley, Calif.: Transform Press, 1997.)

NOTES

CHAPTER 1. SET AND SETTING

1. Murphy, *The Future of the Body*.
2. Lukoff, Zanger, and Lu, "Transpersonal Psychology Research Review."
3. Halpern, "The Use of Hallucinogens in the Treatment of Addiction."
4. Gowan, *Development of the Psychedelic Individual*; Phillips, *The Origins of Intellect*.
5. Winkelman and Roberts, *Psychedelic Medicine*.
6. Goldsmith, "Rescheduling Psilocybin."
7. Rich and Goldsmith, "The Utilization of Policy Research."

CHAPTER 2. IS FUNDAMENTAL PERSONALITY CHANGE POSSIBLE?

1. Marker, "Spritual Emergence" in *The Ecstatic Imagination*.
2. Brightman, "Faith Healer."

CHAPTER 3. THE HISTORY OF PSYCHEDELIC RESEARCH

1. Stoll, "LSD, a Hallucinatory Agent from the Ergot Group."
2. Leary, Litwin, and Metzner, "Reactions to Psilocybin Administered in a Supportive Environment."
3. Henderson and Glass, *LSD*.
4. Doblin, "Reflections on the Concord Prison Experiment and the Follow-up Study," www.maps.org/news-letters/v09n4/09410con.bk.html (accessed August 11, 2010).
5. Dyck, *Psychedelic Psychiatry*.
6. James, *The Varieties of Religious Experience*, 213, footnote.
7. Grinspoon and Bakalar, *Psychedelic Drugs Reconsidered*; Grob, "Psychiatric Research with Hallucinogens"; Grof, *LSD Psychotherapy*; Halpern, "Hallucinogens."

8. Gable, "Toward a Comparative Overview"; Science and Technology Committee, *Classification of Drugs.*

9. Abraham and Aldridge, "Adverse Consequences of Lysergic Acid Diethylamide"; Cohen, "Lysergic Acid Diethylamide"; Halpern and Pope, "Hallucinogen Persisting Perception Disorder"; Halpern and Pope, "Do Hallucinogens Cause Residual Neuropsychological Toxicity?"; Strassman, "Adverse Reactions to Psychedelic Drugs." See also Frecska's 2007 "Therapeutic Guidelines" review of the safety issues in volume one of Winkelman and Roberts' *Psychedelic Medicine* 2007 textbook.

10. Council on Spiritual Practices, *Code of Ethics for Spiritual Guides;* Forte, *Entheogens and the Future of Religion.*

CHAPTER 4. THE TEN LESSONS OF PSYCHEDELIC THERAPY, REDISCOVERED

1. Arthur, *Mushrooms and Mankind;* Devereux, *The Long Trip;* Furst, *Flesh of the Gods;* McKenna, *Food of the Gods;* Weil, *The Natural Mind.*

2. Roberts, *Psychedelic Horizons.*

3. Schultes and Hofmann, *Plants of the Gods.*

4. Narby, *The Cosmic Serpent.*

5. Grob, "Psychiatric Research with Hallucinogens"; Zinberg, *Drug, Set, and Setting.*

6. Dobkin de Rios and Grob, "Hallucinogens, Suggestibility and Adolescence."

7. Pahnke, "LSD and Religious Experience."

8. Yensen, "From Mysteries to Paradigms."

9. Furst, *Flesh of the Gods;* Schultes and Hofmann, *Plants of the Gods.*

10. Badiner, *Zig Zag Zen;* Grinspoon and Bakalar, *Psychedelic Drugs Reconsidered;* Kurland, "LSD in Supportive Care"; Zinberg, *Drug, Set, and Setting.*

11. Pahnke, "The Psychedelic Mystical Experience."

12. Buber, *I and Thou;* Suzuki, *The Sacred Balance.*

13. Dobkin de Rios and Grob, "Hallucinogens, Suggestibility and Adolescence."

14. Zinberg, *Drug, Set, and Setting.*

15. Hofmann, *LSD.*

16. Grof et al., "LSD-assisted Psychotherapy."

17. Stuart, "Psychedelic Family Values."

18. Dobkin de Rios and Grob, "Hallucinogens, Suggestibility and Adolescence"; Grob, "Psychiatric Research with Hallucinogens"; Halpern et al., "Psychological and Cognitive Effects."

19. Stolaroff, "Using Psychedelics Wisely."

20. Furst, *Flesh of the Gods;* Narby, *The Cosmic Serpent.*

21. Huxley, *The Perennial Philosophy.*

22. Council on Spiritual Practices, *Code of Ethics for Spiritual Guides;* Stolaroff, "A Protocol for a Sacramental Service."

23. Council on Spiritual Practices, *Code of Ethics for Spiritual Guides;* Forte, *Entheogens and the Future of Religion.*

24. Furst, *Flesh of the Gods.*

25. Council on Spiritual Practices, *Code of Ethics for Spiritual Guides.*

26. Ibid.

27. Bravo and Grob, "Shamans, Sacraments, and Psychiatrists"; Schultes and Hofmann, *Plants of the Gods.*

28. Stevens, *Storming Heaven.*

29. Furst, *Flesh of the Gods;* Narby, *The Cosmic Serpent;* Schultes and Hofmann, *Plants of the Gods.*

30. Stolaroff, "Using Psychedelics Wisely."

31. Ajaya, *Psychotherapy East and West;* Merkur, *The Ecstatic Imagination.*

32. Ballentine, *Radical Healing.*

33. Smith, "Do Drugs Have Religious Import?"

34. Huxley, *Moksha.*

35. Bateson, *Steps to an Ecology of Mind;* Heard, *The Third Morality;* McTaggart, *The Field;* Teilhard de Chardin, *The Phenomenon of Man.*

36. Murphy, *The Future of the Body.*

37. Ballentine, *Radical Healing.*

38. Ajaya, *Psychotherapy East and West;* Heard, *The Third Morality;* Huxley, *The Perennial Philosophy;* Suzuki, *The Sacred Balance.*

39. McKenna, *Food of the Gods;* Sheldrake, *The Rebirth of Nature;* Wilber, *Integral Psychology.*

40. Ajaya, *Psychotherapy East and West.*

CHAPTER 5. MANY THEORETICAL AND METHODOLOGICAL QUESTIONS REMAIN

1. Grinspoon and Bakalar, *Psychedelic Drugs Reconsidered;* Multidisciplinary Association for Psychedelic Studies, *Psychedelic Research around the World.*

2. Doblin, "The Historic FDA and NIDA Meetings."

3. Stevens, *Storming Heaven.*

4. Shulgin and Shulgin, *PiHKAL.*

5. Barrigar, "The Regulation of Psychedelic Drugs"; Henderson and Glass, *LSD;* Stolaroff, *The Secret Chief;* Strassman, "Human Hallucinogenic Drug Research"; Szasz, *Ceremonial Chemistry;* Weiss, "The Politicization of Evaluation Research."

6. Huxley, *Island.*

7. Merkur, *The Ecstatic Imagination;* Watts, *The Joyous Cosmology.*

8. Wasson, "The Hallucinogenic Fungi of Mexico: An Inquiry into the Origins of the Religious Idea Among Primitive Peoples."

9. Multidisciplinary Association for Psychedelic Studies, "MAPS Protocol #MT-1, Amendment 2: Response to Deferral Letter, December 2, 2009."

10. Grob, *LSD Psychotherapy;* Grof, *Psychology of the Future;* Halpern, "Hallucinogens"; Strassman, "Hallucinogenic Drugs in Psychiatric Research and Treatment."

11. Campbell and Stanley, *Experimental and Quasi-experimental Designs.*

12. Abuzzahab and Anderson, "A Review of LSD Treatment in Alcoholism"; Faillace, Vourlekis, and Szara, "Hallucinogenic Drugs in the Treatment of Alcoholism"; Pahnke and Richards, "Implications of LSD and Experimental Mysticism."

13. Nutt, et al., "Development of a Rational Scale to Assess the Harm of Drugs of Potential Misuse."

14. Kast, "The Analgesic Action of Lysergic Acid."

15. Kast and Collins, "Lysergic Acid Diethylamide as an Analgesic Agent."

16. Kast, "Attenuation of Anticipation."

17. Grof and Halifax, *The Human Encounter with Death;* Grof et al., "LSD-assisted Psychotherapy"; Grof et al., "DPT as an Adjunct"; Kurland, "LSD in Supportive Care"; Pahnke, "The Psychedelic Mystical Experience"; Richards, *Counseling, Peak Experiences and the Human Encounter;* Richards et al., "The Peak Experience Variable"; Yensen, "LSD and Psychotherapy."

18. Pahnke, "The Psychedelic Mystical Experience."

19. Ibid.

20. Phifer, "A Review of the Research."

21. Doblin, "Dr. Leary's Concord Prison Experiment."

22. Hein, "Treatment of the Neurotic Patient."

23. Hein, "Selbsterfahrung und stellungnahme."

24. Abuzzahab and Anderson, "A Review of LSD Treatment in Alcoholism"; Faillace, Vourlekis, and Szara, "Hallucinogenic Drugs in the Treatment of Alcoholism"; Halpern, "The Use of Hallucinogens in the Treatment of Addiction."

25. Halpern et al., "Psychological and Cognitive Effects."

26. Campbell, "Reforms as Experiments."

27. Arthur, *Mushrooms and Mankind;* Devereux, *The Long Trip;* Reidlinger, *The Sacred Mushroom Seeker;* Schultes and Hofmann, *Plants of the Gods;* Weil, *The Natural Mind.*

28. Griffiths et al., "Psilocybin, Mystical-type Experiences."

29. Masters and Houston, *The Varieties of Psychedelic Experience.*

30. Ibid.

31. Pahnke and Richards, "Implications of LSD and Experimental Mysticism."

32. Doblin, "Pahnke's 'Good Friday Experiment': A Long-Term Follow-Up and Methodological Critique."

33. Griffiths et al., "Psilocybin Can Occasion Mystical-Type Experiences Having Substantial and Sustained Personal Meaning and Spiritual Significance."

34. Dobkin de Rios and Janiger, "LSD and Spirituality."

35. Huxley, *The Doors of Perception*, 73.

36. Grof, *LSD Psychotherapy*.

37. Huxley, *Moksha*; Zaehner, *Mysticism*.

38. Porush, "Finding God in the Three-pound Universe."

39. Pahnke and Richards, "Implications of LSD and Experimental Mysticism"; Roberts, *Psychoactive Sacramentals*; Walsh and Grob, *Higher Wisdom*.

40. Ajaya, *Psychotherapy East and West*; Ellwood, *The Sixties Spiritual Awakening*; Wilber, *Integral Psychology*.

41. Center for Cognitive Liberty and Ethics, *Pharmacotherapy*.

42. Council on Spiritual Practices, *Code of Ethics for Spiritual Guides*.

CHAPTER 6. THE DEVELOPMENT OF
AN INTEGRAL CLINICAL PHILOSOPHY

1. Spurgeon, *The Psychospiritual Perspective*.

CHAPTER 7. IMPLICATIONS FOR THE FUTURE

1. Quinn, *Ishmael*; Suzuki, *The Sacred Balance*.

2. Ellwood, *The Sixties Spiritual Awakening*.

3. Wilson, *Consilience*; Hollick, *The Science of Oneness*.

4. Wilber, *Integral Psychology*.

5. Ellwood, *The Sixties Spiritual Awakening*; Horgan, *Rational Mysticism*.

6. Murphy, *The Future of the Body*.

7. Bateson, *Steps to an Ecology of Mind*; Heard, *The Third Morality*; Sheldrake, *The Rebirth of Nature*.

8. Bateson, *Steps to an Ecology of Mind*; Teilhard de Chardin, *The Phenomenon of Man*.

9. Lovelock, *Gaia*.

EPILOGUE

1. Griffiths et al., "Psilocybin Can Occasion Mystical-Type Experiences Having Substantial and Sustained Personal Meaning and Spiritual Significance."

2. Center for Cognitive Liberty and Ethics, *Pharmacotherapy*.

3. Halpern et al., "Evidence of Health and Safety in American Members of a Religion Who Use a Hallucinogenic Sacrament."

4. Strassman, "Human Hallucinogenic Drug Research."
5. Nelkin, "Scientific Knowledge, Public Policy, and Democracy."
6. Ellwood, *The Sixties Spiritual Awakening.*
7. Nutley, Walter, and Davies, *From Knowing to Doing.*

APPENDIX 1. HOW TO PUT SCIENCE INTO ACTION TO CHANGE THE WORLD

1. Beckhard, "Strategies for Large System Change"; Kennis and McTaggart, "Participatory Action Research"; Osborne and Gaebler, *Reinventing Government.*
2. Havelock, *Bibliography on Knowledge Utilization*; Lawler et al., *Doing Research That Is Useful;* Holt, *Implementing Innovation;* Neilson, *Knowledge Utilization;* U.S. Department of Health and Human Services, *Annotated Bibliography.*
3. Barrigar, "The Regulation of Psychedelic Drugs"; McGlothlin, "Social and Para-medical Aspects"; Weiss, "The Politicization of Evaluation Research."
4. Lefebvre, "Theories and Models"; Stern, "Some Observations."
5. Lefebvre, "Theories and Models"; Osborne and Gaebler, *Reinventing Government.*
6. Havelock, *Planning for Innovation;* Paris and Reynolds, *The Logic of Policy Inquiry;* Rich, *The Knowledge Cycle.*
7. Blasiotti, "Disseminating Research Information"; Caplan, "A Minimal Set of Conditions"; Dalziel and Schoonover, *Changing Ways;* Paisley, "Knowledge Utilization."
8. Churchman, *The Systems Approach;* Davenport, *Process Innovation;* Kotter, *Leading Change;* Nutley, Walter, and Davies, *From Knowing to Doing;* Rothman, *Planning and Organizing for Social Change.*
9. Beckhard, "Strategies for Large System Change"; Caplan, "A Minimal Set of Conditions"; Duchnowski, Kutash, and Friedman, *Researchers and Advocates;* Edwards and Gaventa, *Global Citizen Action;* Kennis and McTaggart, "Participatory Action Research"; Paisley, "Knowledge Utilization"; Zaltman, "Knowledge Utilization."
10. Kennis and McTaggart, "Participatory Action Research"; Kotter, *Leading Change;* Lefebvre, "Theories and Models"; Paisley, "Knowledge Utilization."
11. Duchnowski, Kutash, and Friedman, *Researchers and Advocates;* Edwards, "NGOs in the Information Age"; Osborne and Gaebler, *Reinventing Government;* Paisley, "Knowledge Utilization."
12. Blasiotti, "Disseminating Research Information"; Harpignies, *Political Ecosystems;* Kelly, *Out of Control;* Kennis and McTaggart, "Participatory

Action Research"; Nelkin, "Scientific Knowledge, Public Policy, and Democracy."

13. Weiss, "The Politicization of Evaluation Research."

14. Nelkin, "Scientific Knowledge, Public Policy, and Democracy."

15. Argyris, Putnam, and Smith, *Action Science;* Kennis and McTaggart, "Participatory Action Research"; Kotter, *Leading Change.*

16. Duchnowski, Kutash, and Friedman, *Researchers and Advocates;* Edwards and Gaventa, *Global Citizen Action;* Harpignies, *Political Ecosystems;* Rich and Goldsmith, "The Utilization of Policy Research"; Strassman, "Human Hallucinogenic Drug Research"; Weiss, "The Politicization of Evaluation Research."

17. Duchnowski, Kutash, and Friedman, *Researchers and Advocates;* Edwards and Gaventa, *Global Citizen Action.*

18. Ibid.

19. Caplan, "A Minimal Set of Conditions"; Glaser, Abelson, and Garrison, *Putting Knowledge to Use;* Nutley, Walter, and Davies, *From Knowing to Doing.*

20. Blasiotti, "Disseminating Research Information"; Lefebvre, "Theories and Models."

21. Barrigar, "The Regulation of Psychedelic Drugs"; Beckhard, "Strategies for Large System Change"; Caplan, "A Minimal Set of Conditions"; Henderson and Glass, *LSD;* Osborne and Gaebler, *Reinventing Government.*

22. Caplan, "A Minimal Set of Conditions"; Rich and Goldsmith, "The Management and Utilization of R&D."

23. Oskamp, *Attitudes and Opinions;* Schatzman and Strauss, *Field Research;* Selltiz, Wrightsman, and Cook, *Research Methods.*

24. Paris and Reynolds, *The Logic of Policy Inquiry.*

25. Bogdan and Taylor, *Introduction to Qualitative Research Methods.*

26. Kotter, *Leading Change;* Snow, *The Two Cultures.*

27. Blasiotti, "Disseminating Research Information."

28. Weiss, "The Politicization of Evaluation Research."

29. Blasiotti, "Disseminating Research Information"; Caplan, "A Minimal Set of Conditions"; Zaltman, "Knowledge Utilization."

30. Barrigar, "The Regulation of Psychedelic Drugs"; Beckhard, "Strategies for Large System Change"; Center for Cognitive Liberty and Ethics, *Pharmacotherapy;* Churchman, *The Systems Approach;* Edwards and Gaventa, *Global Citizen Action;* Harpignies, *Political Ecosystems;* Rich and Goldsmith, "The Utilization of Policy Research"; Snow, *The Two Cultures;* Weiss, "The Politicization of Evaluation Research."

BIBLIOGRAPHY

Abraham, H., and A. Aldridge. "Adverse Consequences of Lysergic Acid Diethylamide." *Addiction* 88 (1993): 1327–34.

Abuzzahab, F. S., and B. J. Anderson. "A Review of LSD Treatment in Alcoholism." *International Pharmacopsychiatry* 6 (1971): 223–35.

Ajaya, S. *Psychotherapy East and West: A Unifying Paradigm.* Honesdale, Pa.: The Himalayan International Institute of Yoga Science and Philosophy of the U.S.A., 1983.

Argyris, C., R. Putnam, and D. M. Smith. *Action Science.* San Francisco: Jossey-Bass, 1985.

Arthur, J. *Mushrooms and Mankind: The Impact of Mushrooms on Human Consciousness and Religion.* Escondito, Calif.: The Book Tree, 2000.

Assagioli, R. *Transpersonal Development: The Dimension Beyond Psychosynthesis.* London: Crucible/Harper Collins, 1991.

Badiner, A. H., ed. *Zig Zag Zen: Buddhism and Psychedelics.* San Francisco: Chronicle Books, 2002.

Ballentine, R. *Radical Healing: Integrating the World's Great Therapeutic Traditions to Create a New Transformative Medicine.* New York: Three Rivers Press, 1999.

Barrigar, R. H. "The Regulation of Psychedelic Drugs." *The Psychedelic Review* 1, no. 4 (1964): 394–441.

Bateson, G. *Steps to an Ecology of Mind.* Northvale, N.J.: Jason Aronson, Inc., 1987.

Beckhard, R. "Strategies for Large System Change." *Sloan Management Review* 16 (Winter 1975): 43–45.

Blasiotti, E. "Disseminating Research Information to Multiple Stakeholders: Lessons from the Experience of the National Institute on Disability and Rehabilitation Research." Knowledge: Creation, Diffusion, Utilization 13, no. 3 (1992): 305–19.

Bogdan, R., and S. J. Taylor. *Introduction to Qualitative Research Methods: A Phenomenological Approach to the Social Sciences.* New York: Wiley, 1975.

Bravo, G., and C. S. Grob. "Shamans, Sacraments, and Psychiatrists." *Journal of Psychoactive Drugs* 21, no. 1 (1989): 123–28.

Brightman, A. "Faith Healer." *Animal Wellness* 10, no. 1 (February/March, 2008): 54–55; (www.animalwellnessmagazine.com/art/aV101_54.htm. Accessed July 24, 2010.

Buber, M. *I and Thou*. Edinburgh: Clark, 1923.

Campbell, D. T. "Reforms as Experiments." *American Psychologist* 24 (1969): 409–29.

Campbell, D. T., and J. Stanley. *Experimental and Quasi-experimental Designs for Research*. Chicago: Rand McNally and Company, 1967.

Caplan, N. "A Minimal Set of Conditions Necessary for the Utilization of Social Science Knowledge in Policy Formation at the National Level." In *Using Social Research in Public Policy Making*, edited by C. H. Weiss, 183–98. Lexington, Mass.: Lexington Books, 1977.

Center for Cognitive Liberty and Ethics. *Pharmacotherapy and the Future of the Drug War*. Davis, Calif.: Center for Cognitive Liberty and Ethics, 2006.

Churchman, C. W. *The Systems Approach*. New York: Delta Publishing, 1968.

Cohen, S. "Lysergic Acid Diethylamide: Side Effects and Complications." *Journal of Nervous and Mental Disease* 130, no. 1 (1960): 30–40.

Council on Spiritual Practices. *Code of Ethics for Spiritual Guides*. San Francisco: Council on Spiritual Practices 1995; www.csp.org/development/code.html. Accessed August 18, 2010.

Dalziel, M. M., and S. C. Schoonover, eds. *Changing Ways*. New York: American Management Association, 1988.

Davenport, T. H. *Process Innovation*. Cambridge, Mass: Harvard Business School Press, 1993.

Devereux, P. *The Long Trip: A Prehistory of Psychedelia*. New York: Penguin Putnam, 1997.

Dobkin de Rios, M., and C. S. Grob. "Hallucinogens, Suggestibility and Adolescence in Cross-cultural Perspective." *Yearbook of Ethnomedicine* 3 (1994): 113–32.

Dobkin de Rios, M., and O. Janiger. "LSD and Spirituality." In *LSD, Spirituality and the Creative Process*, 115–51. Rochester, Vt.: Park Street Press, 2003.

Doblin, R. E. "Dr. Leary's Concord Prison Experiment: A 34-year Follow-up Study." *Journal of Psychoactive Drugs* 30, no. 4 (1998): 419–26.

———. "The Historic FDA and NIDA Meetings on 'Hallucinogens.'" *Multidisciplinary Association for Psychedelic Studies Bulletin* 3, no. 3 (1992): 2–6.

———. "Pahnke's 'Good Friday Experiment': A Long-Term Follow-Up and Methodological Critique." *Journal of Transpersonal Psychology* 23, no. 1 (1991): 1–28.

Duchnowski, A. J., K. Kutash, and R. M. Friedman. Researchers and Advocates: Silent Partners in Improving the Children's Mental Health System. Lanham, Md.: National Rehabilitation Information Center, 1989.

Dyck, E. Psychedelic Psychiatry: LSD from Clinic to Campus. Baltimore: The Johns Hopkins University Press, 2008.

Edwards, M. "NGOs in the Information Age." IDS Bulletin 25, no. 2 (1994): 117–24.

Edwards, M., and J. Gaventa, eds. Global Citizen Action. Boulder, Colo.: Lynne Rienner, 2001.

Ellwood, R. S. The Sixties Spiritual Awakening: American Religion Moving from Modern to Postmodern. New Brunswick, N.J.: Rutgers University Press, 1994.

Faillace, L. A., A. Vourlekis, and S. Szara. "Hallucinogenic Drugs in the Treatment of Alcoholism: A Two-year Follow-up." Comprehensive Psychiatry 11, no. 1 (1970): 51–56.

Forte, R., ed. Entheogens and the Future of Religion. San Francisco: Council on Spiritual Practices, 2000.

Frecska, E. "Therapeutic Guidelines: Dangers and Contra-indications in Therapeutic Applications of Hallucinogens." In Psychedelic Medicine: New Evidence for Hallucinogens as Treatments, edited by M. Winkelman and T. Roberts. New York: Praeger, 2007.

Furst, P. T., ed. Flesh of the Gods: The Ritual Use of Hallucinogens. New York: Praeger, 1972.

Gable, R. "Toward a Comparative Overview of Dependence Potential and Acute Toxicity of Psychoactive Substances Used Nonmedically." American Journal of Drug and Alcohol Abuse 19, no. 3 (1993): 263–81.

Glaser, E. M., H. H. Abelson, and K. N. Garrison. Putting Knowledge to Use. San Francisco: Jossey-Bass, 1983.

Goldsmith, N. M. "Psychedelics, Psychotherapy, and Change." Video presentation. Psychedelic Science in the Twenty-First Century. San Jose, Calif.: April 16, 2010.

———. A Conversation with George Greer and Myron Stolaroff. Santa Cruz, Calif.: Multidisciplinary Association for Psychedelic Studies, 1998; www.maps.org/secretchief/ggschat.html.

———. "Ethical Standards for Psychedelic Emergencies." 2007; www.cosm.org/goldsmith/ethical.doc.

———. "Fusion of Spirit and Science" (video interview). New York: Postmodern Times, October 27, 2007; www.iclips.net/watch/post-modern-times.

———. "Missed, Mist." Multidisciplinary Association for Psychedelic Studies Bulletin 18, no. 1 (Spring 2008): 35.

———. "Perils and Promise of Entheogens" (video interview). *Entheologue with Alex Grey.* New York: February 29, 2008.

———. "Psychedelic Research: History and Clinical Applications, with Dr. Neal Goldsmith." Video presentation. *Psychedelic and Entheogenic Society of New York City.* New York: August 1, 2009.

———. "Psychology and Psychedelics" (radio interview). *RadiOrbit with Mike Hagan,* Columbia, Missouri: KOPN, 89.5FM, May 12, 2008, www.mike-hagan.com/2012/mp3/051208_NEAL_GOLDSMITH.mp3.

———. "Psychotherapy, Psychedelics, and Change." Video presentation. *Psychedelic and Entheogenic Society of New York City.* New York: April 25, 2009.

———. "Psychotherapy, Psychedelics, and the Emergence of an Integral Society" (radio interview). *Radio Unnamable with Bob Fass.* New York: Pacifica Radio, WBAI, 99.5FM, September 26, 2008.

———. "Psychospiritual Evolution: An Interview with Dr. Neal Goldsmith" (blog interview). *Gnostic Media with Jan Irvin,* Los Angeles: Gnostic Media, May 24, 2009.

———. "The Ten Lessons of Psychedelic Psychotherapy, Rediscovered." In *Psychedelic Medicine: New Evidence for Hallucinogenic Substances as Treatments,* edited by M. Winkler and T. Roberts, vol. 2, 107–41. New York: Praeger, 2007.

———. "Rescheduling Psilocybin: A Review of the Clinical Research." *Affidavit, Municipal/Superior Court of the State of California, County of Santa Cruz,* Case #: S5-04887. December 1995.

———. Review of *LSD: Still with Us after All These Years,* edited by Leigh A. Henderson and William J. Glass. *Multidisciplinary Association for Psychedelic Studies Bulletin* 6, no. 1 (Autumn 1995): 54–57.

Goldsmith, N. M., and J. H. Halpern. "First, Do No Harm." Review of *Harm Reduction Psychotherapy,* by Andrew Tatarsky. *Multidisciplinary Association for Psychedelic Studies Bulletin* 13, no. 1 (Spring 2003): 48–51.

Gowan, J. *Development of the Psychedelic Individual.* Buffalo, N.Y.: Creative Education Foundation, 1974.

Griffiths, R. R., W. A. Richards, U. D. McCann, and R. Jesse. "Psilocybin Can Occasion Mystical-Type Experiences Having Substantial and Sustained Personal Meaning and Spiritual Significance." *Psychopharmacology* 187, no. 3 (2006): 268–83.

Griffiths, R. R., W. A. Richards, M. W. Johnson, U. D. McCann, and R. Jesse. "Mystical-Type Experiences Occasioned by Psilocybin Mediate the Attribution of Personal Meaning and Spiritual Significance 14 Months Later." *Journal of Psychopharmacology* 22, no. 6 (2008): 621–32.

Grinspoon, L., and J. Bakalar. *Psychedelic Drugs Reconsidered.* New York: The Lindesmith Center, 1997.

Grob, C. "Psychiatric Research with Hallucinogens: What Have We Learned?" *Yearbook of Ethnomedicine* 3 (1994): 91–112.

———. "The Use of Psilocybin in Patients with Advanced Cancer and Existential Anxiety." In *Psychedelic Medicine: New Evidence for Hallucinogens as Treatments,* edited by M. Winkelman and T. Roberts. New York: Praeger, 2007.

Grof, S. *Psychology of the Future: Lessons from Modern Consciousness Research.* Albany, N.Y.: SUNY Press, 2000.

———. *LSD Psychotherapy.* Alameda, Calif.: Hunter House, 1994.

Grof, S., L. E. Goodman, W. A. Richards, and A. A. Kurland. "LSD-assisted Psychotherapy in Patients with Terminal Cancer." *International Pharmacopsychiatry* 8 (1973): 129–44.

Grof, S., and J. Halifax. *The Human Encounter with Death.* New York: E. P. Dutton, 1977.

Grof, S., R. A. Soskin, W. A. Richards, and A. A. Kurland. "DPT as an Adjunct in Psychotherapy of Alcoholics." *International Pharmacopsychiatry* 8 (1973): 104–15.

Halpern, J. H. "The Use of Hallucinogens in the Treatment of Addiction." *Addiction Research* 4, no. 2 (1996): 177–89.

———. "Hallucinogens: An Update." *Current Psychiatry Reports* 5, no. 5 (2003): 347–54.

Halpern, J. H., A. R. Sherwood, T. Passie, K. C. Blackwell, and A. J. Ruttenber. "Evidence of Health and Safety in American Members of a Religion Who Use a Hallucinogenic Sacrament." *Medical Science Monitor* 14, no. 8 (2008): SR15–22.

Halpern, J. H., A. R. Sherwood, J. I. Hudson, D. Yurgelun-Todd, and H. G. Pope Jr. "Psychological and Cognitive Effects of Long-term Peyote Use among Native Americans." *Biological Psychiatry* 58, no. 8 (2005): 624–31.

Halpern, J. H., and H. G. Pope, Jr. "Hallucinogen Persisting Perception Disorder: What Do We Know after 50 Years?" Drug and Alcohol Dependence 69, no. 2 (2003): 109–19.

———. "Do Hallucinogens Cause Residual Neuropsychological Toxicity?" *Drug and Alcohol Dependence* 53, no. 3 (1999): 247–56.

Harpignies, J. R. *Political Ecosystems: Modernity, Complexity, Fluidity and the Eco-left.* New York: Spuyten Duyvil, 2004.

Havelock, R. G. *Bibliography on Knowledge Utilization and Dissemination.* Ann Arbor, Mich.: Center for Research on the Utilization of Scientific Knowledge, 1972.

———. *Planning for Innovation through Dissemination and Utilization of Knowledge.* Ann Arbor, Mich.: Center for Research on the Utilization of Scientific Knowledge, 1972.

Heard, G. *The Third Morality*. New York: William Morrow, 1937.

Hein, G. S. A. "Treatment of the Neurotic Patient, Resistant to the Usual Techniques of Psychotherapy, with Special Reference to LSD." *Topical Problems of Psychotherapy* 4 (1963): 50–57.

———. "Selbsterfahrung und stellungnahme eines psychotherapeuten [Self-experience and Statement of a Psychotherapist]." In *Religion und die droge*, edited by M. Josuttis and H. Leuner, 96–108. Stuttgart: Kohlhammer, 1972.

Henderson, L. A., and W. J. Glass. *LSD: Still with Us after All These Years*. New York: Lexington Books, 1994.

Hofmann, A. *LSD: My Problem Child: Reflections on Sacred Drugs, Mysticism, and Science*. Los Angeles: Tarcher, 1983.

Hollick, M. *The Science of Oneness: A Worldview for the Twenty-first Century*. Winchester, U.K.: O Books, 2006.

Holt, K. *Implementing Innovation: An Annotated Bibliography*. Greensboro, N.C.: Center for Creative Leadership, 1987.

Horgan, J. *Rational Mysticism: Dispatches from the Border between Science and Spirituality*. New York: Houghton Mifflin, 2003.

Huxley, A. *The Doors of Perception*. New York: HarperCollins, 2004/1954.

———. *Island*. New York: Harper and Row, 1962.

———. *Moksha: Writings on Psychedelics and the Visionary Experience (1931–1963)*. Los Angeles: Tarcher, 1982.

———. *The Perennial Philosophy*. New York: Harper and Row, 1944.

James, W. *The Varieties of Religious Experience: A Study in Human Nature*. 1902. Reprint, New York: New American Library, 1958.

Johnson, M. W., W. A. Richards, and R. R. Griffiths. "Human Hallucinogen Research: Guidelines for Safety." *Journal of Psychopharmacology* 2 (July 1, 2008): 603–20.

Kast, E. "Attenuation of Anticipation: A Therapeutic Use of Lysergic Acid Diethylamide." *Psychiatric Quarterly* 41 (1967): 646–57.

———. "The Analgesic Action of Lysergic Acid Compared with Dihydro-morphinone and Meperidine." *Bulletin of Drug Addiction Narcotics* 27 (1963): 3517.

Kast, E., and V. Collins, "Lysergic Acid Diethylamide as an Analgesic Agent." *Anesthesia and Analgesia* 43, no. 3 (May–June 1964): 285–91.

Kelly, K. *Out of Control: The Rise of Neo-biological Civilization*. New York: Addison-Wesley, 1994.

Kennis, S., and R. McTaggart. "Participatory Action Research." In *Handbook of Qualitative Research*, edited by N. Denzin and Y. Lincoln. 2nd ed. Thousand Oaks, Calif.: Sage, 2000.

Kotter, J. *Leading Change*. Boston: Harvard Business School Press, 1996.

Kurland, A. "LSD in the Supportive Care of the Terminally Ill Cancer Patient." *Journal of Psychoactive Drugs* 17, no. 4 (Oct.–Dec. 1985): 279–90.

Lawler, E., III, A. Mohrman, Jr., S. Mohrman, G. Ledford, Jr., T. Cummings, and associates. *Doing Research That Is Useful for Theory and Practice.* San Francisco: Jossey-Bass, 1985.

Leary, T., G. Litwin, and R. Metzner. "Reactions to Psilocybin Administered in a Supportive Environment." *Journal of Nervous & Mental Disease* 137, no. 6 (1963): 561–73.

Lefebvre, R. C. "Theories and Models in Social Marketing." In *Handbook of Marketing and Society,* edited by P. N. Bloom and G. T. Gundlach. London: Sage, 2001.

Letcher, A. *Shroom: A Cultural History of the Magic Mushroom.* New York: HarperCollins, 2007.

Lewin, L. *Phantastica, Narcotic, and Stimulating Drugs: Their Use and Abuse.* New York: E. P. Dutton & Company, 1964.

Lovelock, J. *Gaia: A New Look at Life on Earth.* New York: Oxford University Press, 1979.

Lukoff, D., R. Zanger, and F. Lu. "Transpersonal Psychology Research Review: Psychoactive Substances and Transpersonal States." *Journal of Transpersonal Psychology* 22, no. 2 (1990): 107–48.

Masters, R. E. L., and J. Houston. *The Varieties of Psychedelic Experience.* New York: Holt, Rinehart, Janovich, 1966.

McGlothlin, W. H. "Social and Para-medical Aspects of Hallucinogenic Drugs." In *The Use of LSD in Psychotherapy and Alcoholism.* New York: Bobbs-Merrill, 1967.

McKenna, T. *Food of the Gods.* New York: Bantam Books, 1992.

McTaggart, L. *The Field: The Quest for the Secret Force of the Universe.* New York: HarperCollins, 2002.

Merkur, D. *The Ecstatic Imagination: Psychedelic Experiences and the Psychoanalysis of Self-Actualization.* New York: SUNY Press, 1998.

Montagne, M. "Psychedelic Drugs for the Treatment of Depression." In *Psychedelic Medicine: New Evidence for Hallucinogens as Treatments,* edited by M. Winkelman and T. Roberts. New York: Praeger, 2007.

Moreno, F. A., and P. L. Delgado. "Psilocybin Treatment of Obsessive-compulsive Disorder." In *Psychedelic Medicine: New Evidence for Hallucinogens as Treatments,* edited by M. Winkelman and T. Roberts. New York: Praeger, 2007.

Multidisciplinary Association for Psychedelic Studies. "MAPS Protocol #MT-1, Amendment 2: Response to Deferral Letter, December 2, 2009." Santa Cruz, Calif.: Multidisciplinary Association for Psychedelic Studies, 2009; www.maps.org/mdma/mt1_deferral_response_12_02_08.pdf.

———. *Psychedelic Research around the World*. Santa Cruz, Calif.: Multidisciplinary Association for Psychedelic Studies, 2006; www.maps.org/research.

Murphy, M. *The Future of the Body: Explorations into the Further Evolution of Human Nature*. Los Angeles: Jeremy P. Tarcher, 1992.

Narby, J. *The Cosmic Serpent: DNA and the Origins of Knowledge*. New York: Putnam/Tarcher, 1999.

Neilson, S. *Knowledge Utilization and Public Policy Processes: A Literature Review*. Ottawa, Canada: International Development Research Centre, 2001.

Nelkin, D. "Scientific Knowledge, Public Policy, and Democracy." *Knowledge: Creation, Diffusion, Utilization* 1, no. 2 (1979): 106–22.

Nutley, S., I. Walter, and H. Davies. *From Knowing to Doing: A Framework for Understanding the Evidence-into-Practice Agenda*. Discussion Paper 1, Research Unit for Research Utilisation (RURU), University of St. Andrews, Fife, Scotland, and the Network for Evidence-based Policy and Practice, Economic and Social Research Council, Kings College, London, 2002.

Nutt, D., et al. "Development of a Rational Scale to Assess the Harm of Drugs of Potential Misuse." *The Lancet* 369 (March 2007): 1047–53.

Osborne, D., and T. Gaebler. *Reinventing Government*. Reading, Mass.: Addison-Wesley, 1992.

Oskamp, S. *Attitudes and Opinions*. Englewood Cliffs, N.J.: Prentice-Hall, 1977.

Ott, J. *Pharmacotheon: Entheogenic Drugs, Their Plant Sources and History*. Kennewick, Wash.: Natural Products, 1996.

Pahnke, W. "LSD and Religious Experience." In *LSD, Man, and Society*, edited by R. DeBold and R. Leaf. Middletown, Conn.: Wesleyan University Press, 1967.

———. "The Psychedelic Mystical Experience in the Human Encounter with Death." *Harvard Theological Review* 62, no. 1 (1969): 1–32.

Pahnke, W., and W. Richards. "Implications of LSD and Experimental Mysticism." *Journal of Religion and Health* 5, no. 3 (July 1966): 175–208.

Paisley, W. "Knowledge Utilization: The Role of New Communications Technologies." *Journal of the American Society for Information Science* 44, no. 4 (1993): 222–34.

Paris, D. C., and J. F. Reynolds. *The Logic of Policy Inquiry*. New York: Longman, 1983.

Phifer, B. "A Review of the Research and Theological Implications of the Use of Psychedelic Drugs with Terminal Cancer Patients." *Journal of Drug Issues* 7, no. 3 (1977): 287–92.

Phillips, J., Jr. *The Origins of Intellect: Piaget's Theory*. San Francisco: Freeman, 1969.

Porush, D. "Finding God in the Three-pound Universe: The Neuroscience of Transcendence." *Omni* 60 (October 1993): 60–62.

Quinn, D. *Ishmael.* New York: Bantam, 1992.

Rich, R. *The Knowledge Cycle.* Beverly Hills, Calif.: Sage, 1981.

Rich, R., and N. M. Goldsmith. "The Utilization of Policy Research." In *Encyclopedia of Policy Studies,* edited by S. Nagel, 93–115. New York: Marcel Dekker, 1983.

———. "The Management and Utilization of R&D." *Knowledge: Creation, Diffusion, Utilization* 3, no. 3 (1983): 415–36.

Richards, W. *Counseling, Peak Experiences and the Human Encounter with Death: An Empirical Study of the Efficacy of DPT-assisted Counseling in Enhancing the Quality of Life of Persons with Terminal Cancer and Their Closest Family Members.* Ann Arbor, Mich.: University Microfilms, 1975; 75–18, 531.

Richards, W., J. C. Rhead, F. B. DiLeo, R. Yensen, and A. A. Kurland. "The Peak Experience Variable in DPT-assisted Psychotherapy with Cancer Patients." *Journal of Psychedelic Drugs* 9, no. 1 (Jan.–Mar. 1977): 1–10.

Riedlinger, T., ed. *The Sacred Mushroom Seeker: Essays for R. Gordon Wasson.* Portland, Ore.: Dioscorides Press, 1990.

Roberts, T. *Psychedelic Horizons.* Charlottesville, Va.: Imprint Academic, 2006.

———. *Psychoactive Sacramentals.* San Francisco: Council on Spiritual Practices, 2001.

Rogers, E. M. *Diffusion of Innovations.* New York: The Free Press, 1962.

Rothman, J. *Planning and Organizing for Social Change: Action Principles from Social Science Research.* New York: Columbia University Press, 1974.

Schatzman, L., and A. L. Strauss. *Field Research: Strategies for a Natural Sociology.* Englewood Cliffs, N.J.: Prentice-Hall, 1973.

Schultes, R. E., and A. Hofmann. *Plants of the Gods: Their Sacred Healing and Hallucinogenic Powers.* Rochester, Vt.: Inner Traditions, 1992.

Science and Technology Committee. *Classification of Drugs.* Fifth Report of Session 2005–06. London: The United Kingdom Parliament, Science and Technology Committee, 2006; www.publications.parliament.uk/pa/cm200506/cmselect/cmsctech/1031/103102.htm.

Selltiz, C., L. S. Wrightsman, and S. W. Cook. *Research Methods in Social Relations.* 3rd ed. New York: Hold, Rinehart and Winston, 1976.

Sheldrake, R. *The Rebirth of Nature: The Greening of Science and God.* Rochester, Vt.: Park Street Press, 1992.

Shulgin, A., and A. Shulgin. *TiHKAL: The Continuation.* Berkeley, Calif.: Transform Press, 1997.

———. *PiHKAL: A Chemical Love Story.* Berkeley, Calif.: Transform Press, 1993.

Smith, H. "Do Drugs Have Religious Import? A Forty Year Follow-Up." In *Higher Wisdom: Eminent Elders Explore the Continuing Impact of Psychedelics,* edited by R. Walsh and C. Grob. New York: State University of New York Press, 2005.

Snow, C. P. *The Two Cultures and the Scientific Revolution.* New York: Cambridge University Press, 1959.

Stern, H. R. "Some Observations on the Resistance to the Use of LSD-25 in Psychotherapy." *The Psychedelic Review* 2, no. 8 (1966): 105–10.

Stevens, J. *Storming Heaven: LSD and the American Dream.* New York: Harper and Row, 1988.

Stolaroff, M. J. "A Protocol for a Sacramental Service." In *Psychoactive Sacramentals: Essays on Entheogens and Religion,* edited by T. B. Roberts. Santa Cruz, Calif.: Multidisciplinary Association for Psychedelic Studies, 2001.

———. *The Secret Chief.* Santa Cruz, Calif.: Multidisciplinary Association for Psychedelic Studies, 1997.

———. "Using Psychedelics Wisely." *Gnosis* 26 (Winter 1993): 26–30.

Stoll, A. W. "LSD, a Hallucinatory Agent from the Ergot Group." *Swiss Archives of Neurology* 60 (1947): 279.

Strassman, R. "Adverse Reactions to Psychedelic Drugs: A Review of the Literature." *Journal of Nervous and Mental Disease* 172, no. 10 (Oct. 1984): 577–95.

———. "Hallucinogenic Drugs in Psychiatric Research and Treatment." *Journal of Nervous and Mental Disease* 183, no. 3 (1994): 127–37.

———. "Human Hallucinogenic Drug Research in the United States: A Present-day Case History and Review of the Process." *Journal of Psychoactive Drugs* 23, no. 1 (Jan.–Mar. 1991): 29–38.

Stuart, R. "Psychedelic Family Values." *Multidisciplinary Association for Psychedelic Studies Bulletin* 14, no. 2 (Sept. 2004): 47–52.

Suzuki, D. *The Sacred Balance: Rediscovering Our Place in Nature.* Vancouver, Canada: Greystone Books, 1997.

Szasz, T. *Ceremonial Chemistry: The Ritual Persecution of Drugs, Addicts, and Pushers.* Garden City, N.Y.: Anchor Press/Doubleday, 1974.

Teilhard de Chardin, P. *The Phenomenon of Man.* New York: Harper and Row, 1959.

U.S. Department of Health and Human Services. Annotated Bibliography: Information Dissemination to Health Care Practitioners and Policymakers. Bethesda, Md.: U.S. Department of Health and Human Services, 1992.

Walsh, R., and C. Grob, eds. *Higher Wisdom: Eminent Elders Explore the Continuing Impact of Psychedelics.* New York: State University of New York Press, 2005.

Wasson, R. G. "The Hallucinogenic Fungi of Mexico: An Inquiry into the Origins of the Religious Idea Among Primitive Peoples." *Botanical Museum Leaflets* 19, no. 7 (1961). This paper was first given as the Annual Lecture of the Mycological Society of America, Stillwater, Oklahoma, 1960.

Watts, A. *The Joyous Cosmology: Adventures in the Chemistry of Consciousness.* New York: Random House, 1965.

Weil, A. *The Natural Mind.* New York: Houghton Mifflin, 1986.

Weiss, C. H. "The Politicization of Evaluation Research." *Journal of Social Issues* 1 (1972): 37–45.

Weiss, C. H., ed. *Using Social Research in Public Policy Making.* Lexington, Mass.: D.C. Heath and Company, 1977.

Wilber, K. *Integral Psychology: Consciousness, Spirit, Psychology, Therapy.* Boston: Shambhala, 2000.

Wilson, E. O. *Consilience: The Unity of Knowledge.* New York: Random House, 1998.

Winkelman, M. J., and T. B. Roberts, eds. *Psychedelic Medicine: New Evidence for Hallucinogenic Substances as Treatments.* 2 vols. Westport, Conn.: Praeger, 2007.

Yensen, R. "From Mysteries to Paradigms: Humanity's Journey from Sacred Plants to Psychedelic Drugs." In *The Gateway to Inner Space,* edited by C. Rätsch, 11–54. Bridgeport, Conn.: Prism Press, 1989.

———. "LSD and Psychotherapy." *Journal of Psychoactive Drugs* 17, no. 4 (Oct.–Dec. 1975): 267–77.

Zaehner, R. C. *Mysticism: Sacred and Profane.* Oxford: Oxford University Press, 1973.

Zaltman, G. "Knowledge Utilization as Planned Social Change." *Knowledge: Creation, Diffusion, Utilization* 1 (1979): 82–105.

Zinberg, N. E. *Drug, Set, and Setting: The Basis for Controlled Intoxicant Use.* New Haven, Conn.: Yale University Press, 1984.

INDEX